Mindful Beauty

To my parents, Denise and Gilbert,
for their love and my good genes

Editorial Director: Guillaume Robert
Design: Noémie Levain

English Edition

Editorial Director: Kate Mascaro
Editor: Helen Adedotun
Translated from the French by Elizabeth Heard
Copyediting: Wendy Sweetser
Layout Adaptation and Typesetting: Claude-Olivier Four
Proofreading: Nicole Foster
Color Separation: Bussière, Paris
Printed in China by C&C Offset Printing

Originally published in French as *Orahe: Ma Méthode Anti-Âge*
© Flammarion, S.A., Paris, 2016

English-language edition
© Flammarion, S.A., Paris, 2016

editions.flammarion.com

16 17 18   3 2 1

ISBN: 978-2-08-020279-6

Legal Deposit: 12/2016

Estelle Lefébure
With the collaboration of Robert Masson
and Julie Laurent-Marotte

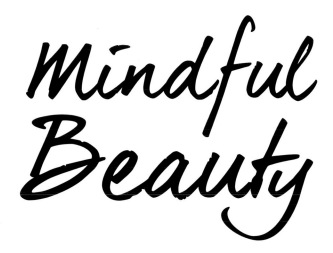

Mindful
Beauty

HOW TO LOOK
AND FEEL GREAT
IN EVERY SEASON

Photographs by Sylvie Lancrenon and Olivier Borde
Recipe photographs by Aline Gérard
Illustrations by Juliette Poney

Flammarion

CONTENTS

Indian Summer 81

Autumn 109

Winter 137

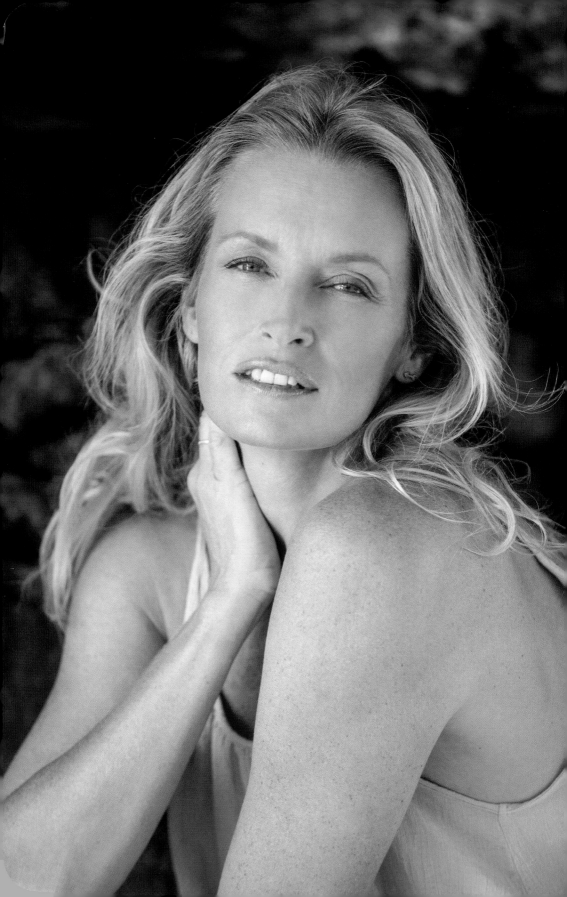

've always aspired to live a healthier, simpler life. Do I want to concentrate on what's truly essential in life? Certainly. Do I want to refocus my energies and take care of other people? Of course I do. Do I want to learn how to listen to the quiet inner voice that tells me what's really best? Naturally.

I've always tried to take care of myself and—over time, with advice from experts—I developed a personal lifestyle program based on health, fitness, well-being, and nutrition. That led me to offer wellness programs under the brand *Orahe*—a Maori word that means health by paddle. As I enter my fifties, I find myself wanting to venture further, using the oar of my paddleboard as the inspiration to explore a new world.

I plan to guide you to the nexus where traditional Chinese medicine, natural healing, and common sense converge. It will be both an enjoyable and a responsible journey, following the gentle rhythm of the passing seasons. You'll learn about a way of life that is mindful of your body and respectful of the planet we live on. It's a healthy approach to living that's accessible to everyone, offering a pathway to gratitude for each moment and a true sense of serenity. ...

"If you choose three passersby at random, one of them will assuredly have something to teach you."

CONFUCIUS

••• I'm not a doctor or a natural healer, so I've drawn extensively on the expertise of specialists such as Robert Masson, founder of the Centre Européen de Naturopathie Appliquée (European Center of Applied Naturopathy), who provides detailed guidance on the relevant health issues in each chapter. When it came to fitness advice, I turned to Julie Laurent-Marotte, coach and sophrology specialist, who helped me design an exercise program for each season.

On the culinary side, in addition to my own creations, I've asked several Michelin starred chefs to devise tasty recipes for us that combine healthy eating with delicious flavors, all using seasonal produce that hasn't spent hours on an airplane to reach our tables.

Are you ready? Welcome aboard on this new journey!

Be *Orahe!*

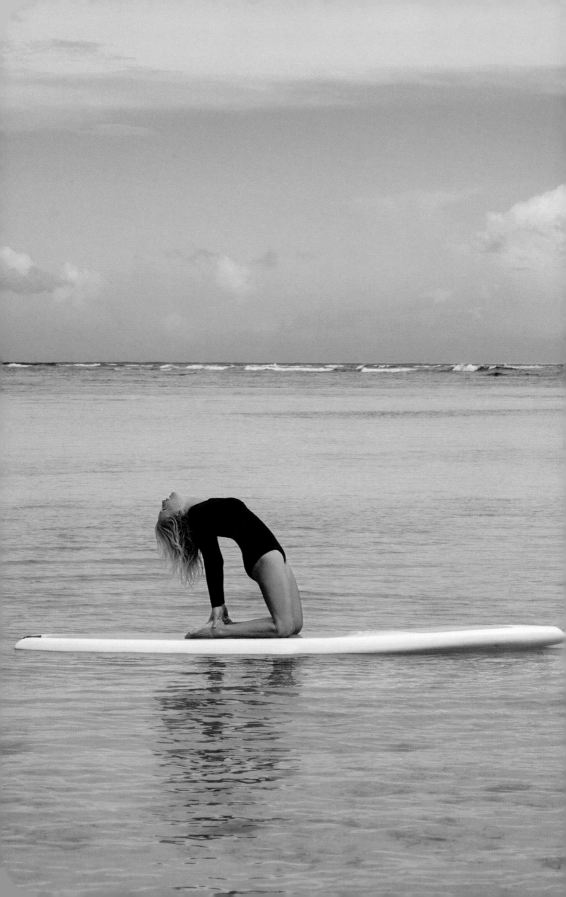

O **health** RA*

+

O **paddle** HE*

=

ORAHE

*in Maori

GENERAL ADVICE

by Robert Masson, naturopathic specialist

Food plays a major role in maintaining the health of our internal organs.

Ideally, we should choose foods that are:
→ **Natural**: free of chemicals, pesticides, preservatives, and artificial colorings
→ **Balanced**: providing all the nutrients required for the body to function healthily
→ **Moderate**: excessive consumption of any type of food can lead to cardiovascular illness, cancer, and a shortened life span
→ **Personalized**: people with a slender build who are sensitive to cold do not have the same requirements as stockier people who always feel warm

So, practically speaking, what should we eat?

Breakfast

For some, this is the most important meal of the day. In winter people who are sensitive to cold should warm up their bodies in the morning. They could try gluten-free cereal flakes (chestnut, rice, buckwheat) cooked with a little almond or other nut butter + a rooibos tea or a tisane spiced with cinnamon or ginger. Or buckwheat pancakes with an egg or a slice of ham + a hot drink. A breakfast like this will fend off those hunger pangs that strike around 11 a.m., helping to maintain a good blood sugar level for the entire day.

Those who are overweight can choose a breakfast based on bananas + nuts + a hot drink (green tea or an infusion, or pure Arabica coffee for those who prefer it).

Lunch

→ Lunch should include seasonal crudités (15–20 % of the meal's weight). Raw vegetables, such as green salad leaves, beets, carrots, celery, fennel, black radish, and Belgian endive, provide beta-carotene and vitamin C (vitamins that are destroyed in cooking), plus minerals and trace elements, as well as the fiber needed for healthy digestion and elimination. People sensitive to cold or those with irritable bowel syndrome should eat these crudités midway through a meal, following a hot main course.

→ An animal protein (meat produced through ethical farming practices that respect animals and the environment), line-caught fish (avoid large fish, which may contain heavy metals), or organic farm-raised eggs, or shellfish (valued for their abundance of trace elements and vitamin B12).

→ A starch (carbohydrate) such as potatoes, sweet potatoes, rice, quinoa, millet, buckwheat, or corn.

→ Cooked green vegetables, particularly for those who want to lose weight or avoid gaining it. Green vegetables are less essential for thin people, but they do provide important fiber and minerals.

→ A dessert is certainly not a health requirement, but it provides an appealing touch of sweetness and satisfaction at the end of a meal. Enjoyed in moderation, it's certainly not harmful. Choose desserts prepared without dairy products or honey. Avoid raw fruit at the end of a meal, but cooked fruit is fine. Why not finish your lunch off with a piece of dark chocolate?

Snack time

It's best to snack on fruits with a high water content around 5:30 p.m. The body has its maximum oxidation capacity at this time of day. Fruit should not be combined with anything starchy (cookies, cereal, etc.), which can result in indigestion and fermentation. The fruit should be eaten alone or with nuts (such as almonds, hazelnuts, walnuts, or cashews), if you're really hungry.

Dinner

Eat sensibly, as you did at lunch. At this meal animal proteins can be replaced by nuts.

Vegetarians can get their protein from eggs or goat or sheep milk cheese.

FOUR VALUABLE TIPS

In addition to eating well, you should also:

→ get regular physical exercise, if only just a half-hour walk each day;

→ get a good night's sleep;

→ keep life's challenges in perspective as much as you can;

→ avoid exposure to electromagnetic waves. You might consider putting an air-purifying Peruvian apple cactus candle by your computer, using a landline rather than a cell phone, and taking a quick shower when you come home from the office.

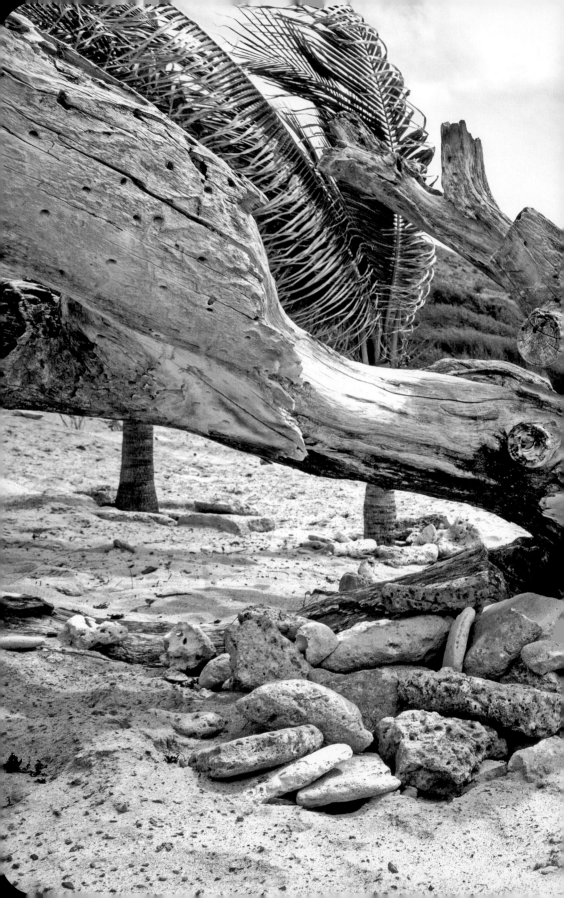

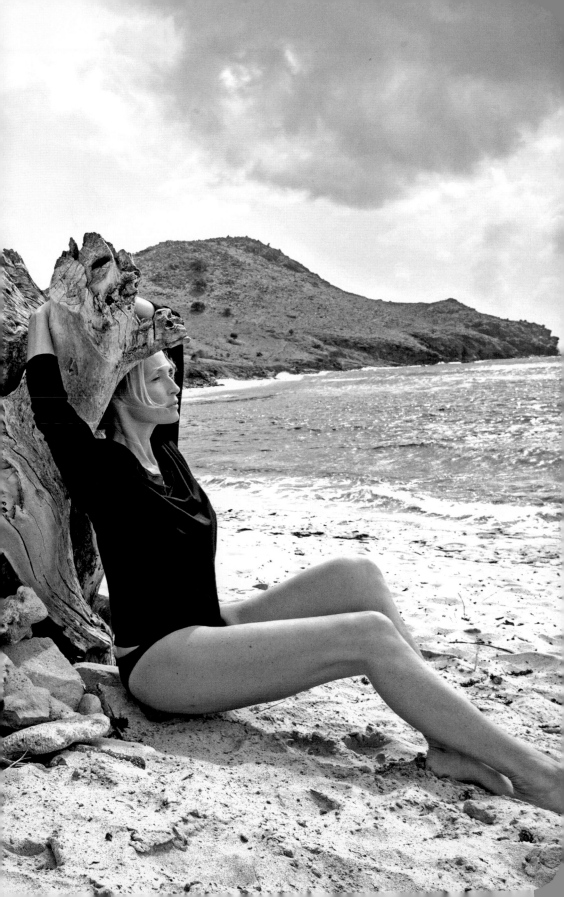

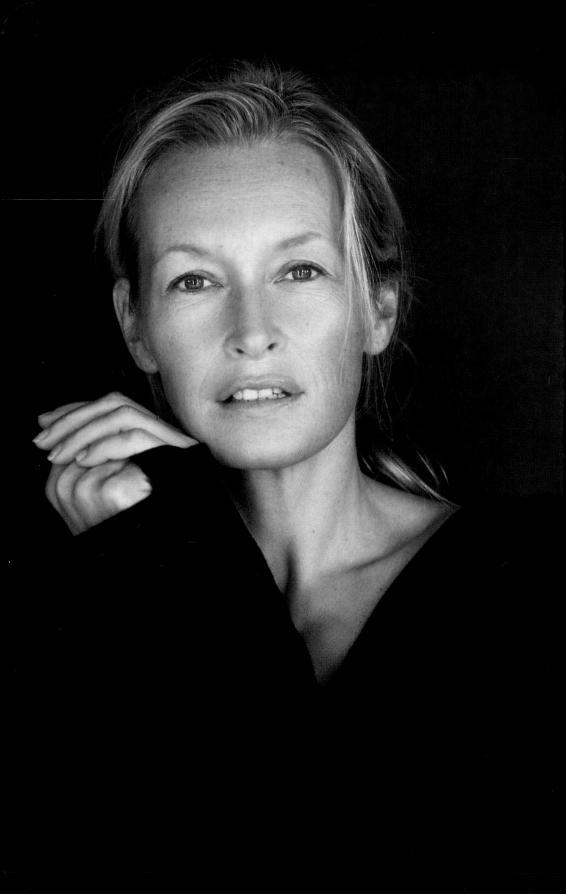

Spring

"Spring: the season of illusions. Nature is rejuvenated and we believe the same to be true of ourselves."

ARISTOTLE

S pringtime is the season of renewal.

As the days lengthen, the first green leaves appear and all of nature seems to reawaken. Spring is often associated with youth, but it is a season of renewal at every age. We can preserve a sense of youthfulness by taking advantage of the surge of energy that rises within us, as sap does within a tree.

In Chinese medicine, spring is the season for paying special attention to the liver, which is often the first organ to give indications of digestive problems. Have you ever noticed that poor digestion can lead to a dull, yellowish complexion? One of the keys to maintaining youthfulness is to understand the factors that can inhibit the liver's functions.

It's well known that industrial products, animal fats, preserved meats, alcohol, and sugary pastries produce acidity and inflammation. But lack of sleep, stress, and anger also adversely affect the liver.

For me, spring is the time to go green. No need to choose between nutritional or spiritual detox as one doesn't work without the other.

Add a fresh touch to your cuisine. Green salads gradually replace hearty soups and beautiful red berries reappear in the market. It's important to follow the cycle of the seasons as much as possible, even though almost every fruit and vegetable is available year-round these days. Admittedly, it's impossible to be a complete locavore in the kitchen, but do try to avoid products that come from the other side of the planet. Visit the farmers' market—it's often less expensive than the grocery store— and get valuable advice from local growers who are familiar with the best producers in your area.

SPRING-CLEANING MY WAY

If you want to feel your best and think clearly, it's important to create a living space that's clean and tidy. Make spring the occasion to carry out a thorough housecleaning, the first step to recovering a sense of control and well-being.

If your drawers are bursting with creased clothes, it's a challenge to choose the day's outfit. If the kitchen cabinets are disorganized, you'll waste time when you're preparing meals. If the children's rooms are cluttered with toys, you're likely to lose patience when doing housekeeping chores. These situations give rise to needless stress.

Obviously you can't expect to get everything arranged and sorted in just one weekend. Take a month and set yourself a goal that's specific and realistic. Go step by step and tackle a new drawer or closet each day. In a few weeks, by spending an hour a day at most, you won't recognize your newly uncluttered interior.

There's an alternative approach that's just as effective—choose a theme. You might decide to work on shoes for a morning. One evening, you could sort socks or toys. And why not consider filling a "piggy bank of dreams" with money raised from selling your cast-off clothes online or holding a garage sale?

Organization is a fine art in Japan. Marie Kondo, the doyenne of "made in Japan" organizational consultation, believes that living in an orderly home has a positive influence on every other aspect of your life. In her best-selling *The Life-Changing Magic of Tidying Up*, she advises getting started by throwing things away. Don't hold back, and retain nothing that doesn't bring you joy.

GIVING

However modest your means, there are always others around you who have less. Don't hesitate to pass along clothes you no longer wear to a friend who admires your sense of style but doesn't have your shopping budget. Do the same with the toys your children have outgrown.

If you're uncomfortable giving things away to friends and neighbors, there are organizations in every community that redistribute and recycle. Find out about them—it's important for other people, for the planet, and for you.

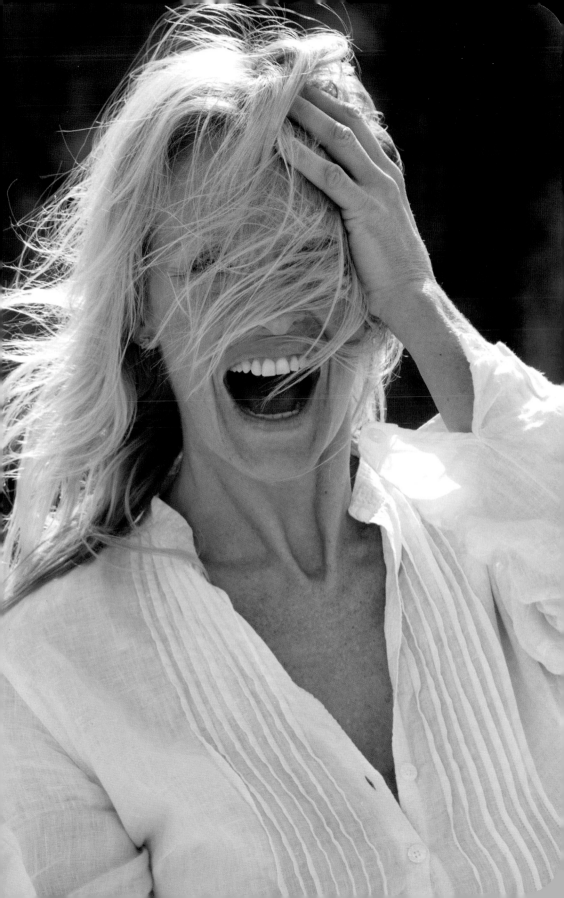

DUST YOURSELF OFF

Standing with my feet the same distance apart as my hips, I close my eyes for a few moments to experience the feeling of my feet in contact with the ground, my bodily sensations, and my breathing. With my eyes open or closed, I press my palms together and rub them until I feel the warmth in my hands, and then I rest them on top of my head. Next, I gently use my fingers and palms to brush away all the imaginary "dust" that I have on me, breathing deeply all the time.

I begin with my hair, eyebrows, eyelids, nose, cheeks, mouth, and ears. Then my neck, shoulders, and arms all the way to my fingertips, the back, chest, stomach, pelvis, hips, buttocks, right leg, left leg, feet, above and below. I take my time while making my movements vigorous and energetic.

Then I roll my back and hold my arms beside my body, combining this movement with deep abdominal breathing. I observe the changes in my bodily sensations, my emotions, my body temperature, my breathing. Doing this exercise in the morning sets you up for a great day.

MY NUTRITIONAL DETOX

While the natural world is rediscovering its vitality, spring is also a good time for us to go green with a personal detoxification program.

These cures have attracted a lot of attention in recent years. They're headlined in magazines and featured in numerous publications. How do you find your way around all this information? Personally, I always prefer simple methods that are accessible and effective. So, in springtime, I consume only vegetable juice or homemade bouillon on one day a week. And I eliminate fat, alcohol, and caffeine for at least three weeks, while eating lots of steamed green vegetables, seasoned with lemon juice, to give my liver function a boost. The evening meal can also be light, replaced by a clear soup. If you fast for more than three days, I recommend professional supervision.

THE LEGENDARY LEMON CURE

After winter's excesses, nothing beats the famous lemon cure—organic lemons, of course, because we use the peel. This cure, which is not a replacement for a meal, is followed for a period of twenty days.

On the first day, boil one lemon, cut in half, for 3 minutes in 2 cups of water. Crush the lemon in the cooking water, then strain. You can drink this beverage throughout the day.

On the second day, use two lemons.

On the third day, three. And so on until the tenth day when you squeeze ten lemons in 2 to 6 cups of water according to taste.

On the eleventh day, cut back to nine lemons. On the twelfth day, use eight. And so on until the last day of the cure.

You'll see from the fresh glow of your complexion that lemon is a wonderful remedy for purifying the liver. Its juice also contributes to the elimination of toxins and fat.

MY SPIRITUAL DETOX

If combined with physical activity, such as brisk walking or swimming, a good nutritional detox should also have a spiritual side. Here are some simple steps to help you shake bad habits and regain your inner radiance:

➜ Rediscover quality sleep by going to bed early
➜ Start a private journal and write in it regularly
➜ Allocate time for quiet reflection
➜ Ignore sensational news coverage and disturbing information
➜ Turn your cell phone off at night
➜ Pay attention to what your dreams are telling you
➜ Take time to enjoy the beauties of the natural world

HUG A TREE

In my opinion, hugging a tree is the very best way to feel at one with nature and draw upon its strength. Find a tree that inspires you, in a garden, park, or forest. Go ahead— clasp your arms around it tightly as if you were lovingly embracing someone dear to you. Press your ear against the trunk to sense its inner life.

Tree hugging may seem odd at first, but it's based on scientific studies. Trees are actually central to our very existence because they convert carbon dioxide into the oxygen that we need every day. So, if we get it at the source, this essential force will have a genuine impact on the stress levels in our minds, as well as the oxygen levels in our tissues.

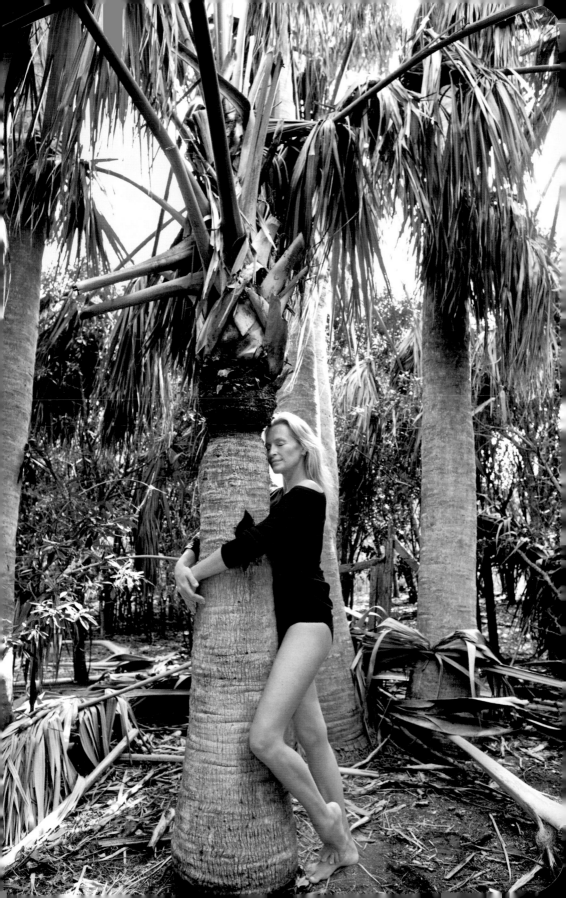

"Trust in grace and the power of transformation."

LYNA JONES

ADVICE FROM A NATUROPATHIC SPECIALIST
FOCUS ON THE LIVER

In springtime, the liver is tired from an excess of fats, alcohol, chocolate, and other winter temptations. If you feel "under the weather," with a sallow complexion and orangey palms, you may be experiencing the effects of a bile deficiency.

What needs to be done to restore this vital organ?

→ Follow the general advice (p. 14)

→ Avoid snacking

→ Limit consumption of dairy products that are laden with growth factors and are currently causing serious health concerns (risk of mastosis, fibroids, etc.)

→ Eat young green vegetables that are very rich in vitamins and minerals. In particular, dandelion greens, which are packed with provitamin A. Also purslane, an excellent liver detoxifier, rich in plant-sourced Omega 3, and which facilitates the development of protective proteins that help repair cellular damage.

→ Use plants that support liver function: desmodium, which is particularly helpful for the after effects of hepatitis, allergies, and headaches; dandelion root for when the complexion is sallow or if you're experiencing lack of appetite or constipation; chrysanthemum (*Chrysantellum americanum*); and artichoke for when cholesterol and triglyceride levels are too high. The plants eliminate these health problems by promoting bile production. Milk thistle is advisable for various forms of liver poisoning caused by heavy metals and drugs. It also has mild hypertension-inducing properties, which can be helpful to those with low blood pressure.

→ At bedtime, place a warm hot-water bottle over the liver. This simple measure will improve its function and, therefore, aid detoxification.

If you've gained a few pounds over the winter, avoid dieting as it does more harm than good over time. To lose those extra pounds, stick to the rule of just one carbohydrate serving per meal. Keep to the general advice, but at lunch and dinner choose either rice, quinoa, buckwheat, millet, potatoes, or sweet potatoes. That's the best way to lose those pounds without depriving yourself, and your health will improve too.

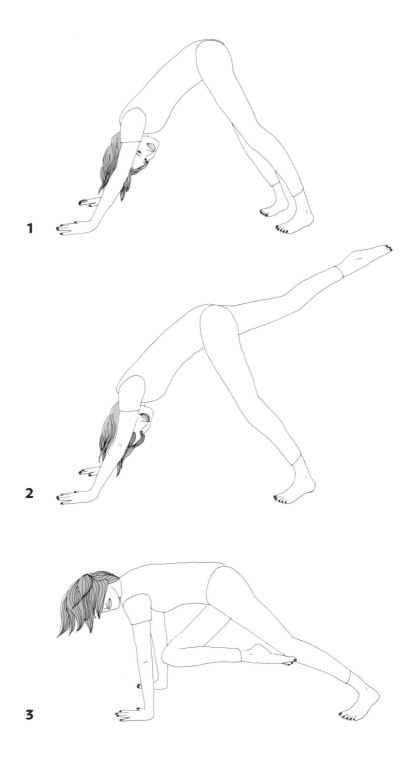

1

2

3

EXERCISES FOR SPRING
THE DOWNWARD DOG

→ Begin by getting down on all fours with your feet flat on the floor. Push your hands against the floor and, using the central abdominal muscles, raise your pelvis upward—you're now in the "downward dog" position. This pose resembles an upside-down V.

→ With every exhalation, bring your chest as close to your thighs as possible, pushing gently down on your hands. Tighten the shoulder blades, let your head hang down, and lower your heels **(1)**.

→ From this position, raise your right leg, keeping it aligned with your back. Contract your buttocks, with your foot stretched out; then flex it—imagine that you're pushing something behind you with your heel **(2)**. Now bring your right knee up to your chest, while simultaneously lowering the hips so that they're parallel with the floor. Your shoulders should be directly above your hands. Pay attention! Do you feel your abdominal muscles coming into play at this exact moment?

→ To take this position to the next level, turn the right knee toward the left elbow as if you're trying to touch them together. Then return the knee to the central axis and raise your right foot backward, pushing down firmly with your hands **(3)**. You'll feel your shoulder muscles working hard.

→ Do at least 5 repetitions per leg, and 3 to 5 sequences.

THE + The "downward dog" enhances blood flow to the brain. This type of position is beneficial to the entire body, but it's especially good for the complexion and the area around the eyes—no more pouches and wrinkles! As for the other merits of this exercise, it strengthens and tones the shoulders and buttocks, and, most importantly, it guarantees you a rock-hard stomach!

HAIR CARE TIPS

The right color

Whether you're a blonde, brunette, or redhead, my top anti-aging hint is to choose the right hair color. Avoid shades that are too dark or uniform—these can add years to you. The most becoming color will be intense and radiant, with complementary tones that create attractive highlights. But stay away from rainbow color hair dyes— they are rarely flattering!

My favorite products

Famous Parisian stylist Christophe Robin has looked after my hair for years. I've even heard rumors that some of his clients ask for "Estelle's blonde." Fact or fiction? I wonder. Among the products offered by this truly brilliant artisan-colorist, I'm a wholehearted fan of his Intense Regenerating Balm with Rare Prickly Pear Seed Oil. It's a complete hair and body care product that you can take with you anywhere. For blondes, I also recommend the Brightening Hair Finish Lotion with Fruit Vinegar, which restores radiance to your hair and provides continuing protection. And if I want to feel like I'm vacationing at the beach all year round, I just spritz on Franck Provost's Styling Ocean Spray: Effet Plage or Bumble and Bumble Surf Spray.

My homemade hair treatments

Banana honey masque: if you've run out of your favorite hair care product in the bathroom, and your hair seems dry or dull, just take a little detour to your kitchen for a solution to your problem. Mash a banana, add 3 tablespoons of honey, and a few drops of sweet almond oil—that's all you need! Apply to hair and wait about 30 minutes, then lather with your usual shampoo.

Another idea: you can try an application of 100 % pure organic argan oil before every shampoo.

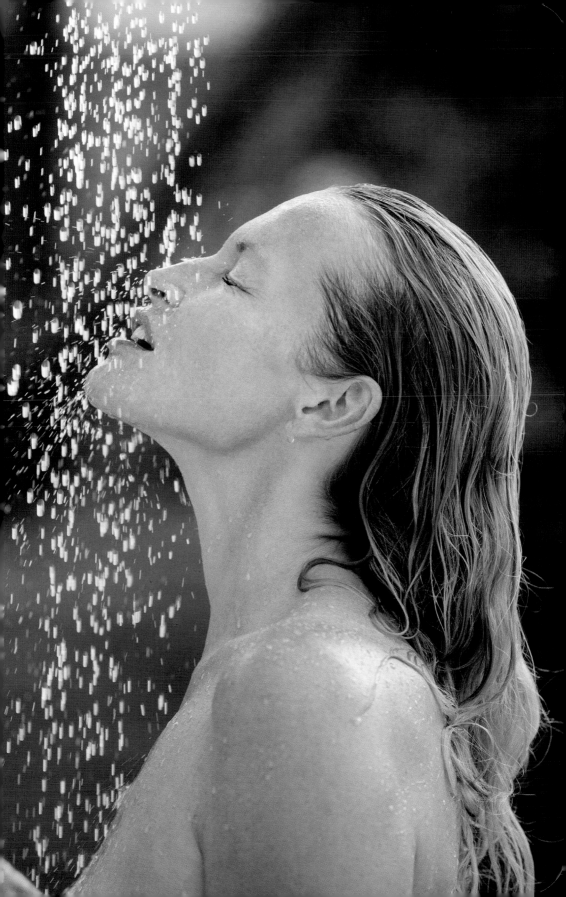

My seasonal market basket

Fruits
Apples
Cherries
Kiwi fruit
Pears
Rhubarb
Strawberries

...

Vegetables
Artichokes
Asparagus
Beets
Cabbages
Carrots
Cauliflower
Celery
Cucumber
Eggplants
Endives
Green peas
Leeks
Lettuces
Onions
Potatoes
Radishes
Spinach
Zucchini

...

ARTICHOKES

Artichokes are grown during the winter months and are among the first spring vegetables to come to market. Native to the Mediterranean region, the artichoke is a member of the cardoon family. The Greeks and Romans valued its leaves and flowers for their medicinal properties.

Rich in antioxidants, including various phenolic and anthocyanoin components, the artichoke is first and foremost an excellent source of nutritional fiber. Insoluble fiber helps to prevent cardiovascular illness. Soluble fiber helps digestion and regularity. For providing minerals and trace elements, the artichoke is a good source of magnesium, iron, copper, phosphorus, zinc, and calcium. It also contains inulin, a non-digestible sugar classified as a prebiotic, which gives the vegetable its distinctive sweetness. Very low in caloric density, despite its high carbohydrate content, it is highly valued in weight loss programs for its satiating effects. My favorite variety is the Brittany artichoke, steamed for 30 minutes and served with good vinaigrette. In Provence, purple baby artichokes are enjoyed *à la barigoule,* when they are fried gently in olive oil and white wine, together with carrots, garlic, and onion.

My Vinegar-Free Vinaigrette
1 tablespoon olive oil
1 tablespoon canola oil
Juice of ½ lemon
1 teaspoon honey
1 pinch of kosher salt
Whisk all the ingredients together until evenly combined.

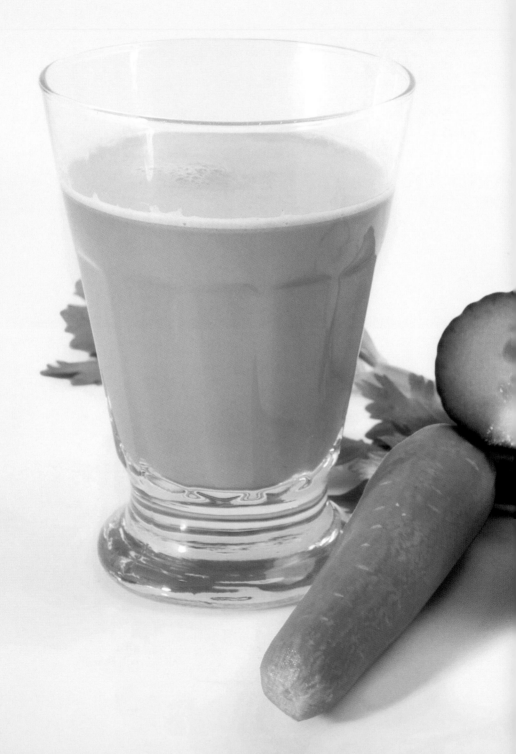

Bikini Juice

Serves 2

Ingredients
1 apple, peeled and
    quartered
2 large carrots, cut into
    pieces
2 celery stalks
½ cucumber, peeled and
    cut in half
½ organic lemon
½ cup (1 oz./25 g) parsley,
    chopped
2 tablespoons vegetable
    protein powder (e.g.
    hemp, raw brown rice,
    soybean)
1 piece of fresh ginger,
    grated

To prepare the juice
Put the fruits and vegetables through
a juicer. Add the chopped parsley,
vegetable protein powder, and grated
ginger to taste.

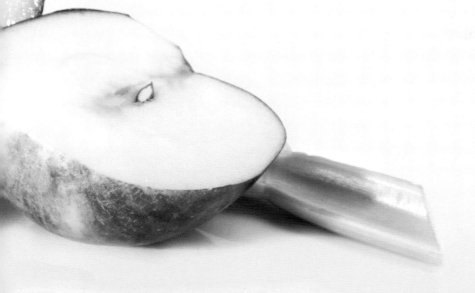

Super Spring Rolls

Serves 2

Ingredients
For the spring rolls
3 large carrots
2 asparagus stalks
1 bunch of fresh mint
2 or 3 avocados, peeled and
   pitted
4 rice spring roll wrappers
9 oz. (250 g) soybean
   sprouts
A few radish sprouts

For the sauce
Juice of 1 lemon
6 teaspoons honey
1 teaspoon tamari soy sauce
½ teaspoon maca powder
1 shallot, peeled
1 teaspoon mixed white and
   black sesame seeds
1 pinch of red beet powder

To prepare the rolls
Wash the carrots, asparagus, and mint. Cut the carrots, asparagus, and avocado into julienne strips. Lay a rice wrapper on a plate and dampen with a little warm water to soften it. Wipe with paper towel before arranging one quarter of the raw asparagus, carrots, soy sprouts, mint leaves, and radish sprouts on top. Roll up the wrapper tightly around the filling, folding over the end to close the roll. Repeat for the other three wrappers and the rest of the filling. Chill for about 1 hour 30 minutes.

To prepare the sauce
Combine the lemon juice, honey, and tamari sauce in a bowl. Add the maca powder and whisk in. Put the shallot through a garlic press and add it to the mixture, along with the sesame seeds and beet powder. Stir together and store in a cool place.

Arrange two rolls on each plate and serve with a small bowl of sauce.

Bon appétit!

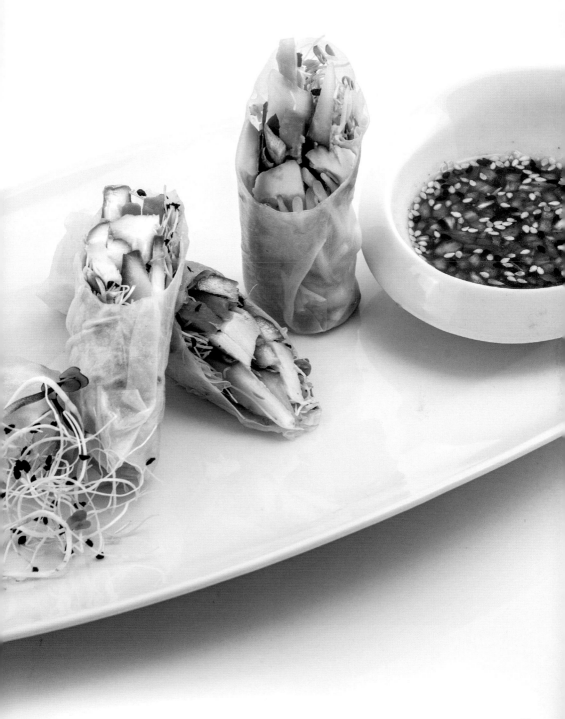

Ilona's Vitamin-Rich Salad

My daughter Ilona adores this colorful salad.

Serves 1

Ingredients
For the cashew nuts
2 tablespoons tamari soy
   sauce
1 tablespoon organic honey
Pepper
2 handfuls of cashew nuts

For the salad
5 carrots
Juice of 1 lemon
Curry powder
1 handful of raisins
Fresh cilantro leaves,
   very finely chopped
Grated fresh coconut
1 slice of lemon, cut into
   6 pieces

For the vinaigrette
2 tablespoons olive oil
1 teaspoon organic cider
   vinegar

To prepare the cashew nuts
Put the tamari, honey, and pepper in a skillet over high heat. When the mixture is hot, add the cashews and cook for a few minutes, stirring. Remove from the heat when the nuts are well caramelized.

Spread out the cashews on a sheet of parchment paper and allow to cool.

To prepare the salad
Wash and grate the carrots and place in a bowl. Sprinkle with lemon juice and a little curry powder.

Add the raisins, caramelized cashews, chopped cilantro, grated coconut, and lemon pieces.

To prepare the vinaigrette
Combine the olive oil and cider vinegar. Dress the salad with the vinaigrette and toss before serving.

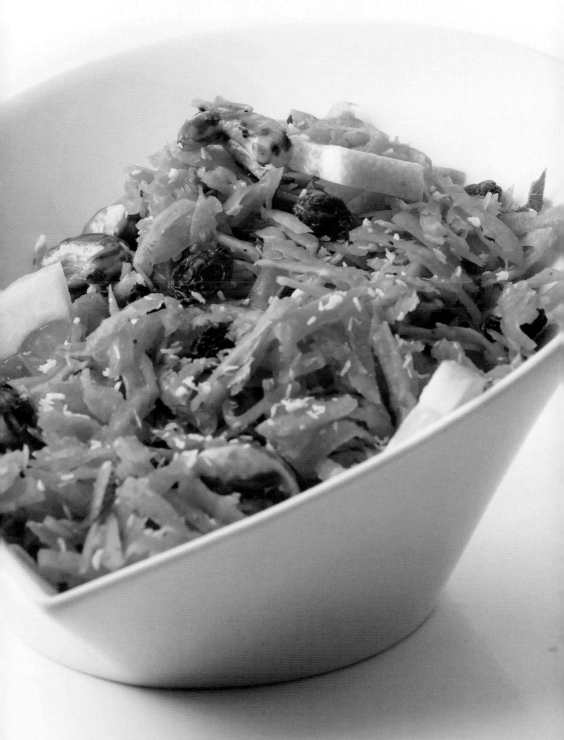

Holy Mackerel!

<u>Serves 1</u>

Ingredients
For the sauce
1 teaspoon lime juice
1 teaspoon tahini
2 teaspoons honey
1 pinch of salt

For the salad
½ red onion, peeled
½ avocado, peeled
   and pitted
½ lemon
A few arugula leaves
A few cooked kidney beans
2 mackerel fillets, skinned
A few soybean sprouts
A few alfalfa seeds
1 handful of pine nuts
2 thin slices of lime

<u>To prepare the sauce</u>
Combine all the ingredients in a bowl.

<u>To prepare the salad</u>
Cut the red onion, avocado, and lemon into thin slices.

Arrange the arugula in a wide shallow bowl and scatter over the slices of onion and avocado, and the kidney beans.

Arrange the two mackerel fillets in the middle of the salad. Add the soybean sprouts, alfalfa seeds, and a few pine nuts. Finally add the two thin slices of lime.

Pour the sauce over just before serving.

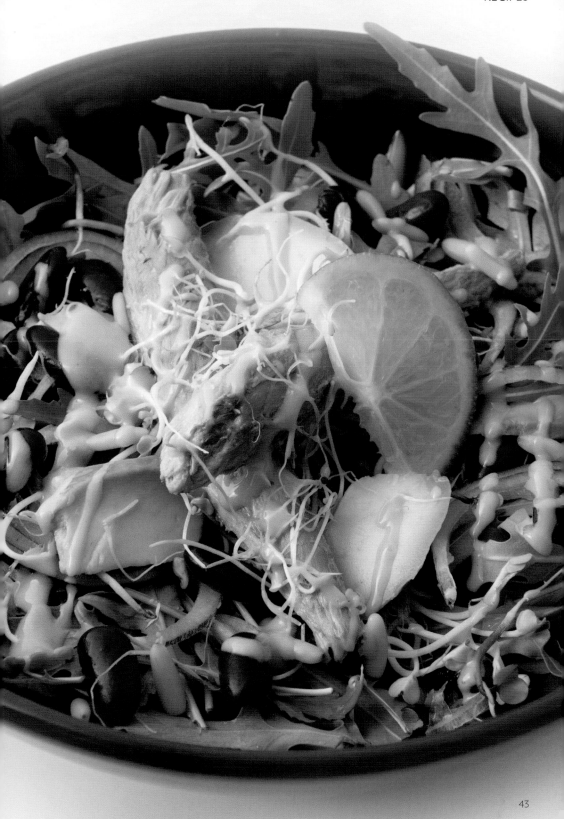

Recipe from David Faure
Aphrodite restaurant, Nice

Pea Gazpacho with Minted Snow Eggs, Spring Vegetables, Soft-Boiled Quail Eggs, and Bottarga

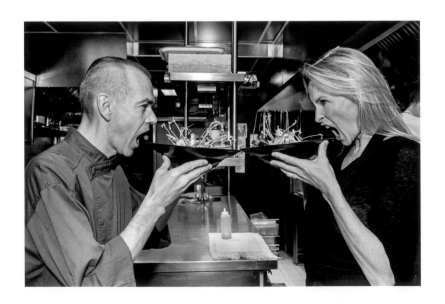

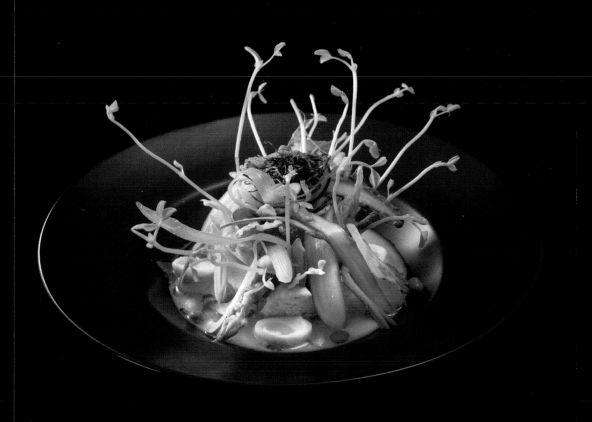

Serves 4

Ingredients

1 lb. (500 g) fresh peas,
   shelled
½ white onion, peeled
   and very finely chopped
Citrino olive oil
4 basil leaves, slivered
1 pinch of ground *piment
   d'Espelette*
4 egg whites
5 fresh mint leaves, slivered
10 quail eggs
8 carrot tops
5 green asparagus stalks
5 white asparagus stalks
1 fennel bulb
1 bunch of pink radishes
1 yellow zucchini or
   1 trumpet zucchini
2 Italian scallions
3 ½ oz. (100 g) pea shoots
16 fresh almonds
½ oz. (15 g) olive oil caviar
Raspberry wine vinegar
1 oz. (30 g) bottarga
Fine salt and kosher salt
Freshly ground pepper

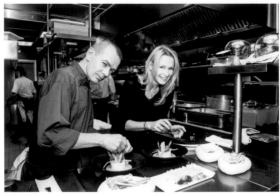

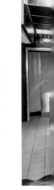

To prepare the ingredients

Blanch the peas in salted boiling water for 90 seconds. Drain, reserving the cooking liquid, and refresh the peas in ice water to preserve their bright green color. Set 2 tablespoons of the peas aside. Marinate the remaining peas for 1 hour with the white onion, olive oil, slivered basil, *piment d'Espelette,* and 2 ladles of the cooled cooking liquid. Season with salt and pepper. Set the remaining cooking liquid aside.

Blend the peas and put them through a sieve. Adjust the seasoning and dilute with a little cooking liquid if the gazpacho seems too thick. Set aside and chill.

Beat the egg whites with a pinch of salt until they hold soft peaks, then add the slivered mint and a generous splash of Citrino olive oil. Using two spoons, form four evenly sized quenelles on a plate covered with plastic wrap, and microwave on full power for 15 seconds or until the quenelles are set. Set aside and chill.

Cook the quail eggs for 2 minutes in barely simmering water. Drain, cool them,

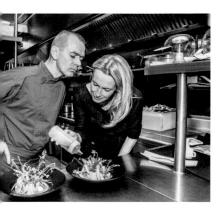

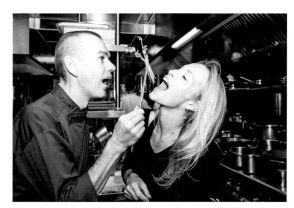

and remove the shells. Cut them in half, being careful not to let the yolks run. Set aside and chill.

Blanch 2 carrot tops, 2 green asparagus stalks, and 2 white asparagus stalks in boiling water, keeping them slightly firm. Drain and refresh in ice water. Cut all the other vegetables into very fine slices and plunge them into ice water so they curl up and crisp.

To serve
Spoon 2 ladles of the gazpacho into well-chilled shallow dishes and top each one with an egg-white quenelle. Season the sliced vegetables, the cooked vegetables, and the peas with Citrino olive oil, wine vinegar, kosher salt, and freshly ground pepper. Arrange all the ingredients attractively, building them up in the center (imagine you are creating a floral arrangement), and finish with the quail eggs, fresh almonds, pea sprouts, olive oil caviar, grated bottarga, and a generous splash of Citrino olive oil for the final glistening touch.

CHEF'S TIPS

→ **You can substitute frozen peas for fresh—there are excellent-quality frozen products available.**

→ **Consider adding toasted croutons just before serving to give crunch and a pleasing contrast of textures.**

→ **The vegetables in this ultra-fresh starter can be adjusted according to market offerings and seasonal availability. A few nasturtium flowers would be a welcome addition for their slightly peppery flavor.**

→ **As a variation and to save time, you can replace the egg-white quenelles with a generous dollop of fresh goat cheese or even silken tofu.**

You get the idea—use the basic recipe as inspiration to create your own unique interpretation.

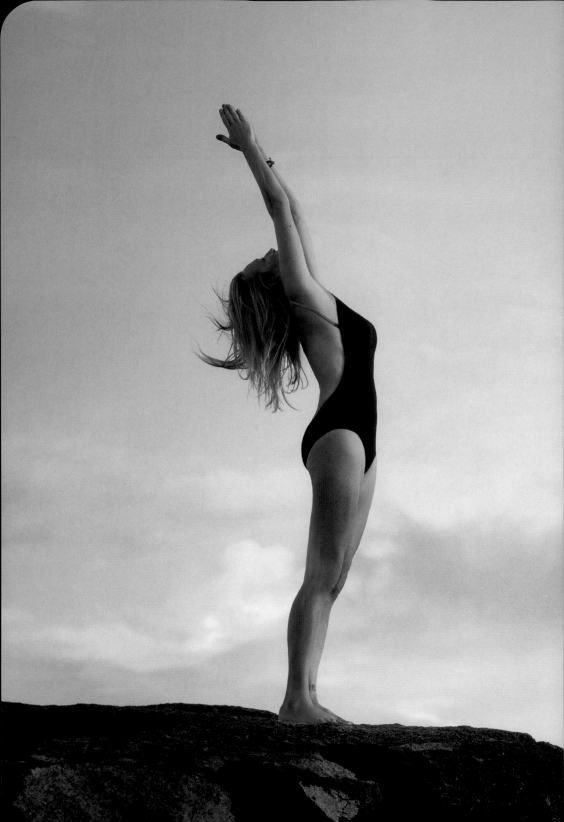

Summer

"Summer: the time when we take our time."

ARISTOTLE

S ummer is the season of vibrant energy. Gardens are in full flower and the warmth of the sun penetrates our hearts and bodies. Often associated with vacations, summer is the season when it is important to set aside time to live in the moment and delight in all these days have to offer.

Chinese medicine considers summer to be the season when special attention is paid to the heart, both physically and emotionally. Our skin is the outward manifestation of heart health. A flushed complexion is often a sign of an emotional state that is close to anger. Pallor suggests anemia or even a state of shock.

For living and aging well, nothing is better than a healthy heart. Once again, sound nutrition has a tremendous impact on the quality of our blood. Beware of very rich dishes containing an excess of animal fats. If you find yourself suffering from low energy levels, choose lighter foods. Don't fall prey to draconian diet regimes—just eat properly; it can make you feel young again.

As the warm weather returns, beware also of excessive indulgence in things such as alcohol, tobacco, and barbecued meats, which can be harmful to cardiac health.

I always make sure that I'm well hydrated during the summer months, and I try to make the most of every moment.

So why not learn how to be happy?

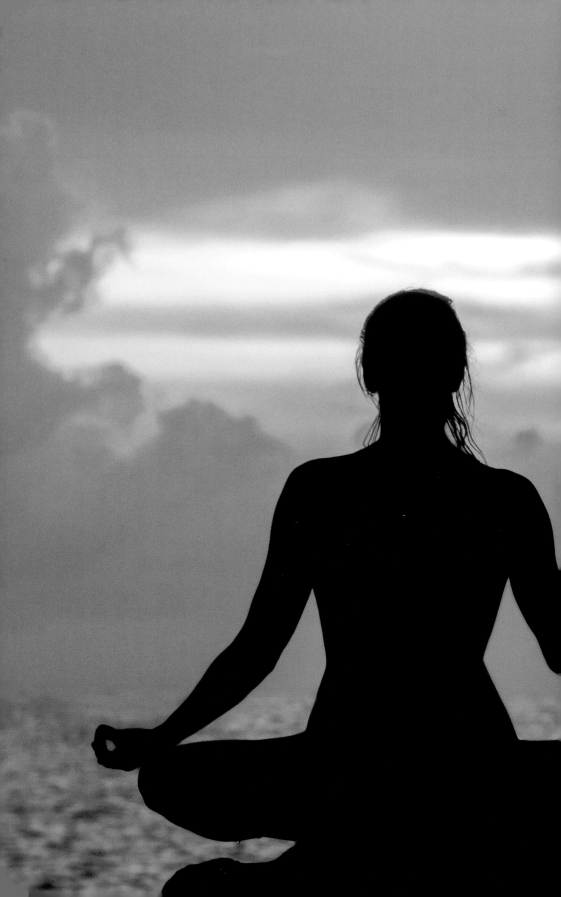

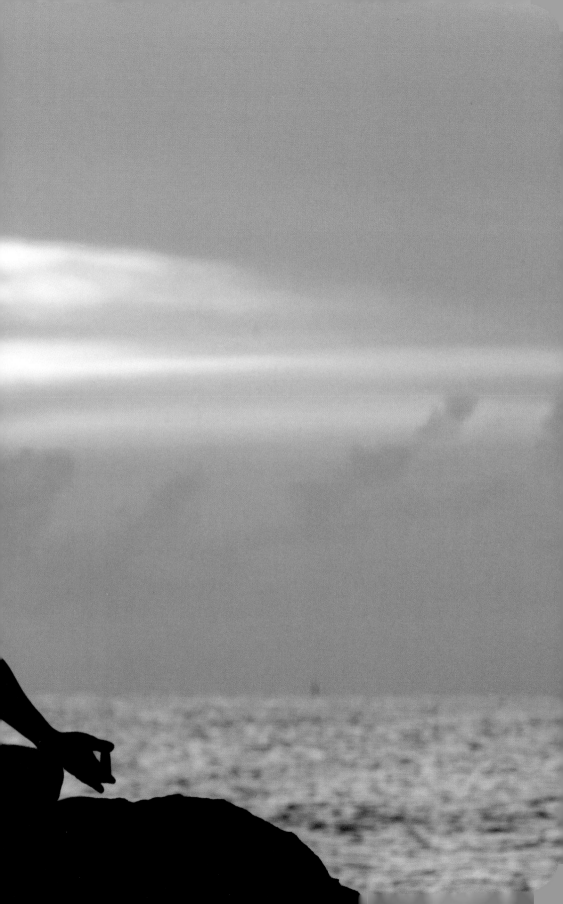

BE OPEN-MINDED

Summer is the season when you can open up your mind to others, to nature, and to yourself. It's a time to listen, share, and give.

Everything seems to happen too fast in modern life. Take advantage of long summer days to cultivate compassion toward others. Take time to listen closely to friends and family, as well as to new acquaintances who come your way.

It's also an opportunity to put your whole heart into your activities and make the most of every minute. Are you genuinely relishing every good meal that's served to you or that you've patiently prepared? Are you really listening to your favorite music without letting yourself be distracted? Are you truly appreciating the beautiful landscapes before you? A shady forest, a field of sunflowers, shimmering reflections in a lake.

Sometimes it's important to do something for others and expect nothing in return. Simple spontaneous acts, like offering a sincere compliment, or telling a close friend how much she means to you. Why not pay for the coffee that your neighbor at the next table just ordered? These are simple acts of kindness whose sole purpose is to give a little happiness to others. Use this summer to break down the walls you've built around yourself.

Open up!

WALK BAREFOOT

It's easier to reconnect with nature when the weather's lovely outside. Put your shoes away on evenings and weekends and let your feet experience a breath of fresh air. Did you know that putting your feet in contact with the earth has a calming effect and helps you recover your sense of equilibrium? What's more, it helps the body rid itself of all those electromagnetic waves emitted by the cell phones and computers that surround us every day. It goes without saying that your open-air strolls should be enjoyed without those online accessories! Take the chance to revive all of your senses: listen to birdsong, breathe in the fresh air, contemplate the skies, savor a wild berry, feel the rough bark of a tree.

Ten ways to generate good vibrations

Offer a compliment

Encourage someone close to you

Offer to buy a stranger a coffee

Tell your friends how much you really care

Wear a t-shirt with a positive message

Give someone a smile without expecting one back

Read for pleasure

Dance to your favorite summer hit

Give yourself a break

Above all, don't feel guilty

MY ANTI-DIET

Don't expect me to reveal my top model diet tips. I don't
have any and I never have. Frankly, I am pretty much
against dieting.

Professionally, I've had the good fortune of belonging to
a generation of models with curvaceous figures, at a time
when young girls weren't pushed toward anorexia.

These days, if I find I've gained extra pounds, I simply eat
a bit less and exercise a bit more. The pounds you might be
able to lose with a draconian diet will always come back.

THE CELERY CURE

Celery is summer's brightest culinary star and you can eat
it all day long. As leaves or seeds, raw as a nibble with
an aperitif, cooked as a side dish for fish, juiced for
a hydrating refresher, or in soup for a light meal, celery is
rich in antioxidants. It even has anti-inflammatory effects
and is beneficial in the treatment of high blood pressure.

Did you know that the ancient Egyptians gathered celery
seeds and stalks to use for seasoning? And if you toast
celery seeds for a few minutes in a skillet, without any oil,
they'll give your soups and salads a delicious fragrance.

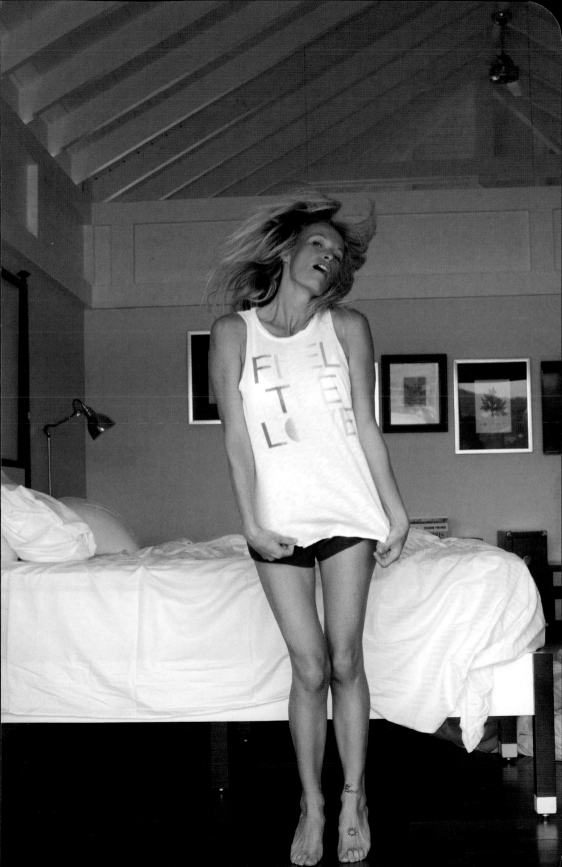

ADVICE FROM A NATUROPATHIC SPECIALIST
FOCUS ON THE HEART

While healthy people aren't affected by heat waves, others can suffer from fatigue and exhaustion or, by contrast, experience nervous agitation that can lead to disturbed sleep.

If you experience fatigue, make sure you take a nap after lunch. Rest facilitates digestion and enhances overall vitality. A brief walk in the shade is also a good idea.

You can enhance your energy level by applying two or three drops of black spruce *(Picea mariana)* extract to the lower back when you wake up.

People who experience the opposite effect from heat—nervous tension and overstimulation—should limit their consumption of caffeinated beverages (coffee, tea, chocolate, tea-based drinks, guarana, etc.). Before bedtime, apply two drops of lavender *(Lavandula angustifolia)* to the inside of the elbow along with two drops of ylang-ylang essential oil.

The heart has to work harder during the summertime to circulate the blood, and the return of venous blood is sometimes less efficient. The legs, particularly between the ankles and knees, can become slightly swollen with a sensation of heaviness, and the capillaries and veins may be more visible. There are a number of plant-based remedies for this condition. Butcher's broom, sweet clover, horse chestnut, and common grapevine all encourage good blood circulation, but our preference leans toward the buds of the ash, chestnut, or horse chestnut trees.

During the summer months, diminished sleep time, increased outdoor activities, and heat combine to make greater demands on the heart. You should therefore avoid overburdening the cardiac system by taking a few simple precautions, avoiding:
➜ overexposure to heat: try not to stay out, exposed and inactive, for too long, especially when the sun is at its peak;
➜ strenuous exercise: engage in gentler activities, like walking in the water or swimming;
➜ activities after meals that inhibit the digestive process: it's a good idea to take a nap;
➜ consuming excess calories. Increase your consumption of raw vegetables (25–30 % of the total meal) and, without making any other changes, try to choose either a starch or a dessert for each meal. Do the same with alcohol. Don't drink more than one glass of wine with your evening meal. If the combination of fatigue and heat causes mild cardiac arrhythmia, take ten drops of the highly effective hawthorn bud extract, which regulates the heartbeat, each morning and evening.

During the summer, lemons and other citrus fruits help stockier, ruddy-skinned people, who prefer cold weather and meat-based meals, to cope with the heat. Drinking the juice of one or two lemons at 5:30 p.m. is excellent for their health.

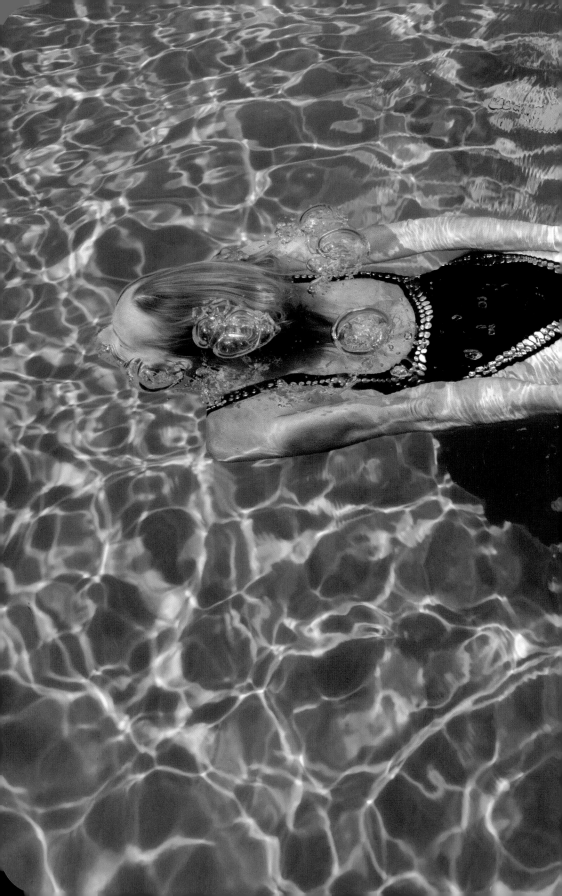

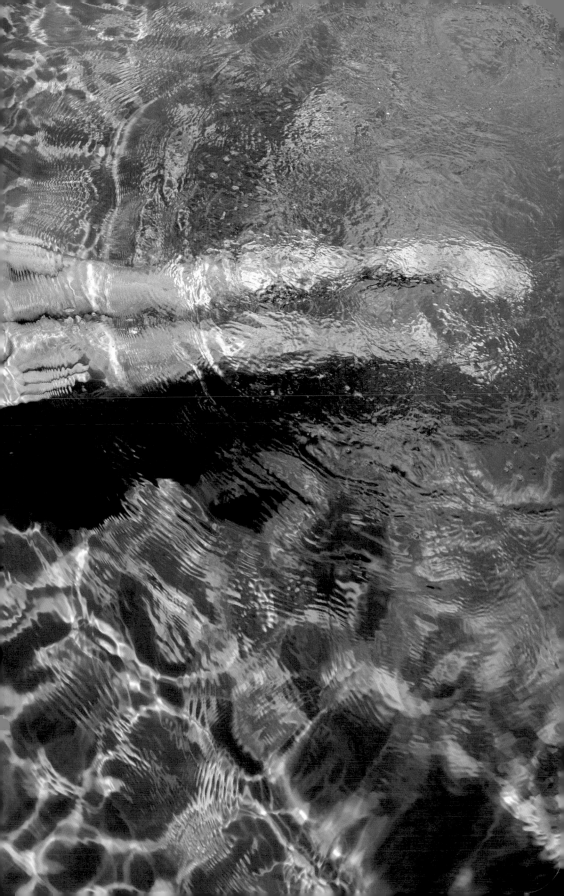

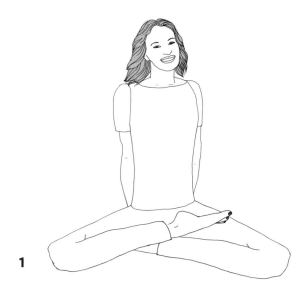

1

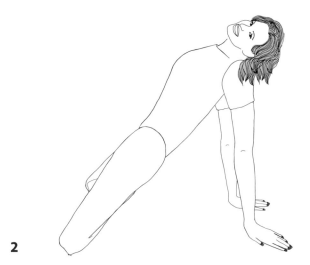

2

EXERCISES FOR SUMMER
SEATED POSITION WITH SHOULDERS PULLED BACK

→ Sit comfortably on your exercise mat in the lotus position (cross-legged) and rest the tips of your fingers on the floor behind your buttocks. As you breathe in, pull your shoulders back, raise your chin, and look up **(1)**. If you'd like to take this position to the next level, raise your buttocks off the floor, contracting them slightly, and open out your thighs and hips to create space between your vertebrae **(2)**.

→ When exhaling, gently rest your buttocks on the floor and return to a seated position, keeping your back straight. Then place your hands in front of you on the floor and walk your fingers forward as far as possible, with your body and head following, so you have forward flexion, bringing your body and head as close as possible to the floor. Take 5 deep breaths in this position. Then roll your back, vertebra by vertebra, using your hands on the floor to support yourself, and return to the starting position.

→ These two exercises complement each other. The seated position with shoulders pulled back gently corrects your posture, and opens out the solar plexus and body core. The forward flexion allows the vertebrae to be stretched out, opens out the lower body, and calms the mind.

→ Repeat these movements at least 3 times, every day, and you'll soon have posture fit for a queen.

THE + At the end of this exercise, be aware of your breathing and the opening and stretching of your diaphragm and abdominal muscles. Try to maintain this overall posture throughout the day. Observe and record your progress. With regular practice, you'll add a few millimeters—or even a few centimeters—to your height, and you'll carry yourself more gracefully.
   Don't give up—you'll be justifiably proud of yourself if you persevere!

BODY CARE TIPS

Genuine Marseille soap

Genuine unscented Marseille soap is the *ne plus ultra* for bathing. It's more ecologically sound, more economical, and altogether healthier and hypoallergenic, too. A bar of Marseille soap will last you almost a month, if it's high quality. But do make sure you're not being cheated as 95 % of what's sold in stores is fake. Check the label carefully for your soap's source and ingredients. My favorite soap maker is Fer à Cheval in Marseille, with its attractive horseshoe logo (www.savon-de-marseille-boutique.com).

Hydration

Your skin needs daily moisturizing after you shower, especially if you want to preserve a youthful complexion. I've been using Mixa's moisturizer for years now, as well as Cattier's body milk with coconut butter and vanilla, both of which are available online. Eucerin Daily Replenishing Moisturizing Lotion is also great. When returning from my own little paradise, I always bring back Idalmi St. Barth Vitamin E Body Spray. You can add fragrance to it with any of your favorite essential oils. It's my idea of magic, whether you use it to moisturize your skin or perfume your linen. It's available online too (idalmistbarth.com/en)!

Ecological exfoliation

I have a little vacation beauty secret that's available to all, at no extra cost! When I'm lucky enough to spend a couple of hours on a beach with lovely fine sand, I take the opportunity to exfoliate naturally. All you have to do is rub a handful of sand over your body, paying extra attention to areas with rough skin, such as the elbows, knees, and heels. And nothing beats a dip in the ocean to rinse off afterwards.

My sugar exfoliant

Mix 2 tablespoons of liquid coconut oil with raw sugar until it has the consistency of a paste. It's an exfoliant with a delightful fragrance that works for the entire body. An anti-aging tip for the face is to add 1 teaspoon of loose green tea to the mix.

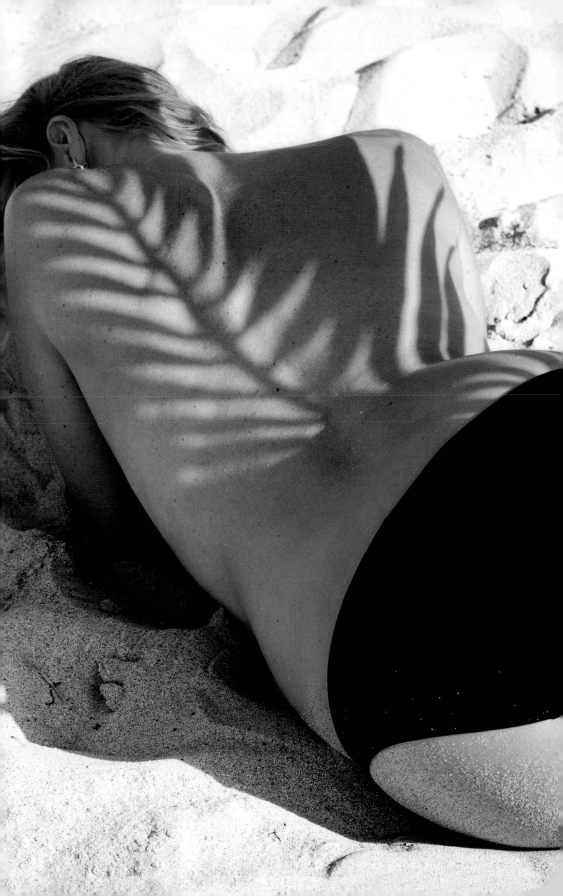

My seasonal market basket

Fruits
Apples
Apricots
Blackberries
Blueberries
Cherries
Figs
Gooseberries
Grapes
Melons
Nectarines
Peaches
Pears
Plums
Raspberries
Rhubarb
Strawberries
...

Vegetables
Artichokes
Asparagus
Beets
Bell peppers
Broccoli
Carrots
Cauliflowers
Celery
Cucumbers
Eggplants
Fennel
Green beans
Green peas
Lettuces
Onions
Potatoes
Radishes
Spinach
Tomatoes
Zucchini

...

FIGS

Originally from Asia, figs are the iconic summer fruit. They've been cultivated all around the Mediterranean since the time of the ancient civilizations. The Egyptians, Phoenicians, Greeks, and Romans all ate figs and revered the tree that bore them.

Rich in antioxidants, including phenolic components from the flavonoid family, figs have so much nutrition in their skins that I recommend they be eaten unpeeled. They're also a great source of soluble and insoluble fiber. Among the minerals and trace elements they provide, figs contain an abundance of potassium, iron, and copper, as well as B vitamins. From June until late August, French markets offer two major varieties: white and purple (the latter contain a higher concentration of antioxidants). When fresh figs are no longer in season, don't hesitate—especially if you're an athlete—to eat dried figs as these offer a higher level of quality nutrients than other dried fruits, such as raisins and dates. Figs go well in all kinds of recipes, sweet or savory. I often use them in summer salads, but they also pair very well with goat or sheep milk cheeses.

My Fig Jam
2 lb. (1 kg) figs
⅓ cup (80 ml) liquid honey
1 vanilla bean
Juice of 1 lemon

Wash and stem the figs, keeping the skin intact, then dice them. Macerate the figs for a day with the honey and vanilla. Cook for 30 minutes over medium heat, stirring regularly. Add the lemon juice and stir one last time before pouring into jars.

THE SEASON FOR JUICE

Summer is the season when market stalls display the widest variety of fruits. Make sure you choose organic produce, especially if you're going to eat the skin, and try to buy from local growers.

Use your juicer to indulge your creative impulses. Invent your own blends, always making sure to include a vegetable among the ingredients to limit the beverage's sugar content. Avoid orange juice before breakfast on an empty stomach— it impedes healthy digestion.

Jus de Provence

Here is a deliciously simple drink
that will give you a peachy glow.

Serves 1

Ingredients
½ cup (120 ml) almond milk
5 strawberries, halved
1 peach, pitted and cut into
    quarters
Lavender flowers

To prepare the juice
Pour the almond milk into a blender. Add the halved strawberries, the peach quarters, and a few lavender flowers. Blend until smooth. Serve in a tall glass with a few extra lavender flowers sprinkled on top.

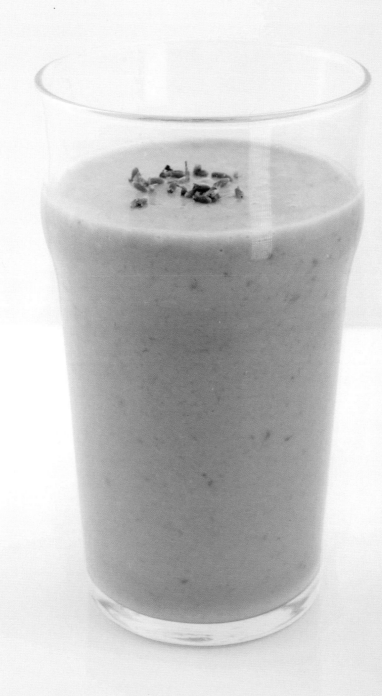

"Déjeuner sur l'Herbe" Salad

Serves 6

Ingredients
For the salad
3 ½ oz. (100 g) arugula
6 oranges, peeled and sliced
3 mangoes, peeled and flesh
   sliced
10 strawberries, sliced
6 small Persian cucumbers,
   sliced
3 raw Chioggia beets, sliced
10 radishes, sliced
2 very ripe avocados, peeled,
   pitted, and chopped
6 tablespoons fresh herbs
   (mint, basil, and cilantro),
   washed and finely chopped

For the sauce
4 limes, squeezed
4 tablespoons olive oil
2 teaspoons agave syrup
1 green chili, sliced
1 teaspoon salt
1 teaspoon freshly ground
   pepper

To prepare the salad
Arrange a generous handful of arugula on a serving platter. Cover with layers of the fruits and vegetables, alternating the colors for a pleasing effect.
Top the salad generously with most of the avocado and herbs.

To prepare the sauce
Combine all the ingredients, except the green chili, and spoon over the salad. Finish by scattering over the remaining avocado, herbs, and the sliced chili.

You can serve this salad with grilled chicken or homemade guacamole.

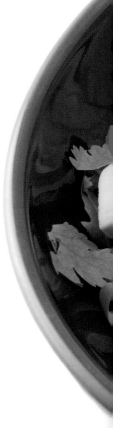

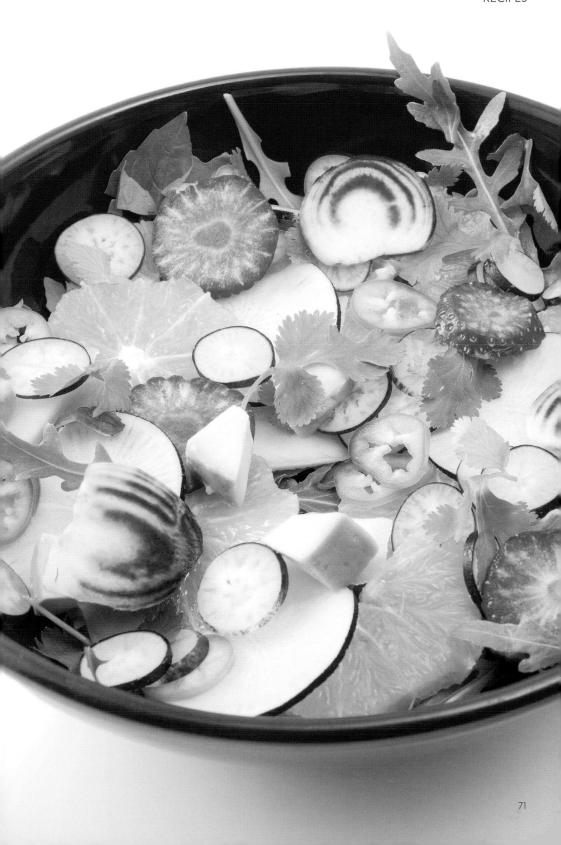

Quinoa-Roq Salad

Serves 4

Ingredients
For the vinaigrette
2 oz. (50 g) walnut halves,
  lightly toasted
1 garlic clove, peeled and
  finely chopped
2 oz. (50 g) watercress
2 tablespoons red wine
  vinegar
1 teaspoon Dijon mustard
Grated zest of 1 orange
4 tablespoons olive oil
Salt and freshly ground
  pepper

For the salad
12 oz. (330 g) quinoa,
  cooked and browned
  in a skillet
2 beets, cooked and sliced
2 oz. (50 g) Roquefort
  cheese, crumbled
Salt and freshly ground
  pepper

To prepare the vinaigrette
Chop the walnuts and add to the garlic. Transfer this garlic-nut mixture to a bowl. Chop the watercress finely and add to the bowl together with the vinegar, mustard, and orange zest. Stir to combine. Gradually pour in the olive oil, whisking constantly. Add salt and pepper to taste.

To prepare the salad
Divide the quinoa equally between four shallow dishes or bowls. Cover each portion of quinoa with an equal amount of beets. Sprinkle the beets with the crumbled Roquefort. Mix the vinaigrette thoroughly and pour 2 or 3 tablespoons over each salad. Serve immediately.

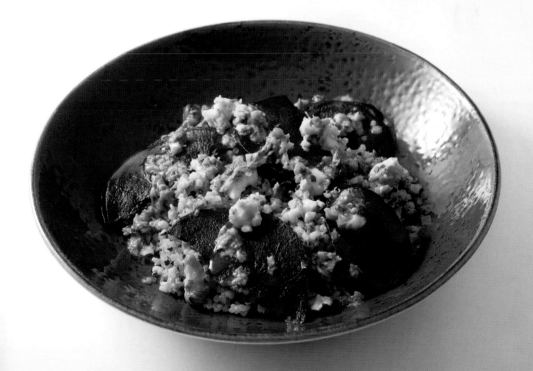

Summertime Pizza Surprise

My son Giuliano adores snacking on this healthy treat.

Serves 6

Ingredients
½ watermelon, sliced
6 strawberries
1 small container
   of blueberries
2 kiwi fruit
1 peach
1 banana
Grated coconut

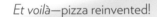

To prepare the pizza surprise
Cut the watermelon slices into triangles.
Wash the strawberries and blueberries.
Peel the kiwis, peach, and banana.
Cut all of the fruit, except the
blueberries, into slices. Arrange the cut
fruit on the watermelon pieces,
to resemble a traditional pizza. Sprinkle
with grated coconut.

Et voilà—pizza reinvented!

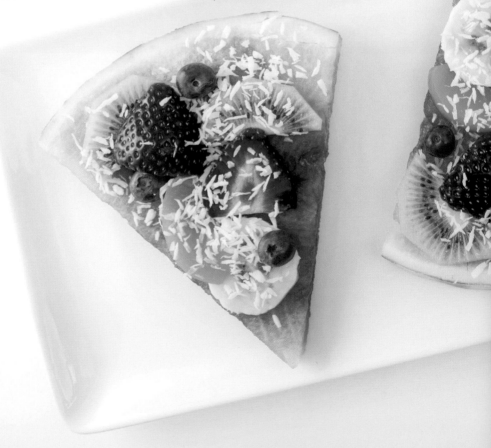

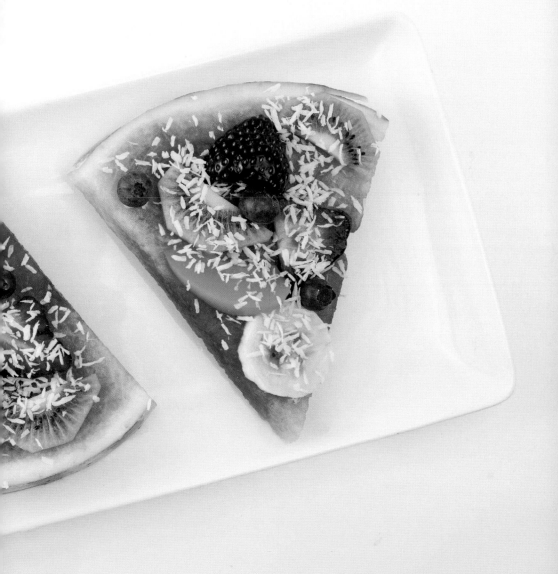

Recipe from Éric Fréchon
Céleste restaurant at
The Lanesborough hotel,
London, and Epicure
restaurant at Le Bristol hotel,
Paris

Chilled Cucumber and Coconut Milk Soup

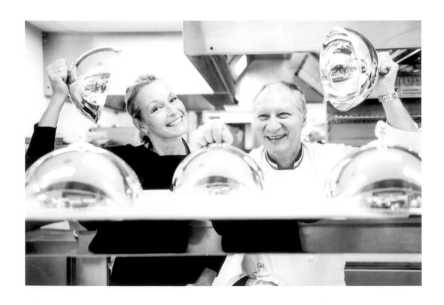

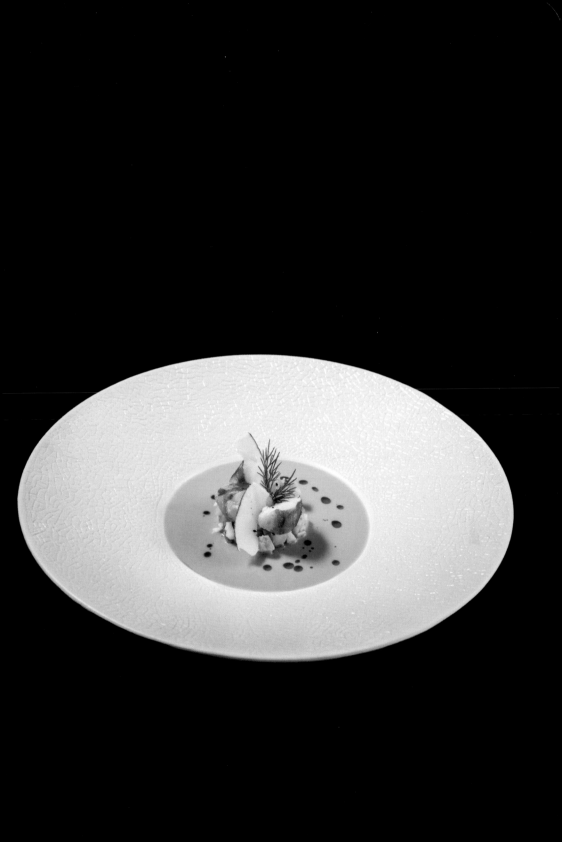

Serves 6

Ingredients
3 medium cucumbers
3 tablespoons olive oil
1 can (14 fl. oz./400 ml)
    coconut milk
1 pinch of curry powder
Kosher salt
Fine salt

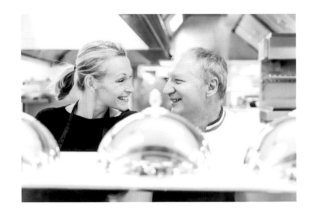

To prepare the soup
Bring a saucepan of water seasoned with kosher salt to a boil.

Peel the cucumbers, taking care to preserve their peel. Cut the cucumbers into large cubes.

Open the can of coconut milk.

Once the water has come to a boil, blanch the cucumber peel for 3 minutes. Drain and refresh immediately in ice water. Drain the peel again and refrigerate.

Pour the olive oil into another saucepan. Add the cucumber cubes, the coconut milk, and the curry powder. Cook over very low heat for 7 minutes.

Put all the ingredients in a blender, not forgetting the cucumber peel as it will give the soup a lovely green color.

Adjust the seasoning, adding salt and extra curry powder to taste.

Strain the soup through a fine-mesh sieve to make it very smooth with no lumps remaining. Refrigerate the soup for at least 2 hours. Serve well chilled.

CHEF'S TIP

→ **You can serve this soup with a garnish of chopped crabmeat.**

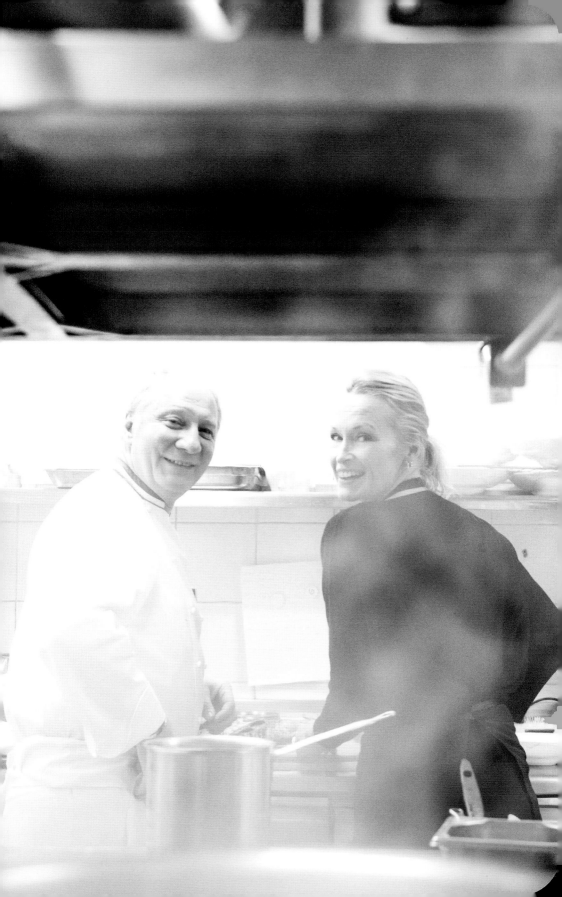

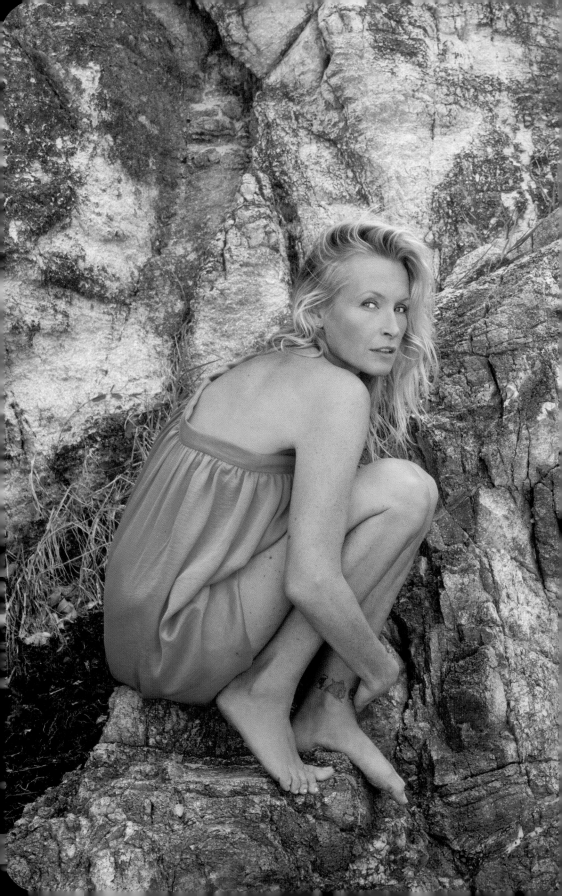

Indian Summer

"It was that rare kind of autumn day that you only find in North America. Over there, they call it Indian summer."

LYRICS TO "INDIAN SUMMER"
BY JOE DASSIN

While we usually refer to the four seasons of the year, there is a bonus season that allows the glow of summer to last a little longer. What North Americans call an Indian summer is known as an "old ladies' summer" in Germany, a "little quince summer" in Spain, an "All Saints' summer" in Sweden, and a "fern summer" in Brittany, France, in honor of the fronds that turn red at this time of year.

Indian summer is a time of transition. Warm weather lingers, and we enjoy the last outdoor meals of the season. But nature is entering a new cycle. Another school year begins, and as parents we strive to help our children overcome challenges and learn patience.

Chinese medical tradition tells us that at this time of year we should pay particular attention to the stomach, an organ that's akin to a food processor, undergoing constant change. Its health, and that of the spleen, is important in avoiding digestive acidity. Don't consume excessive amounts of acidic foods and be careful with spices that may irritate the stomach. And, above all, make sure you chew thoroughly! It's a simple piece of advice, but synonymous with good health.

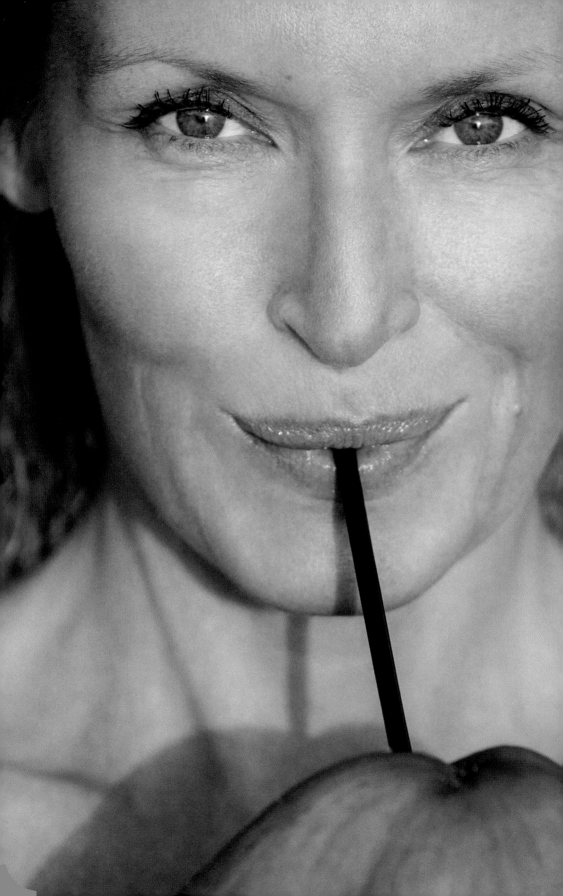

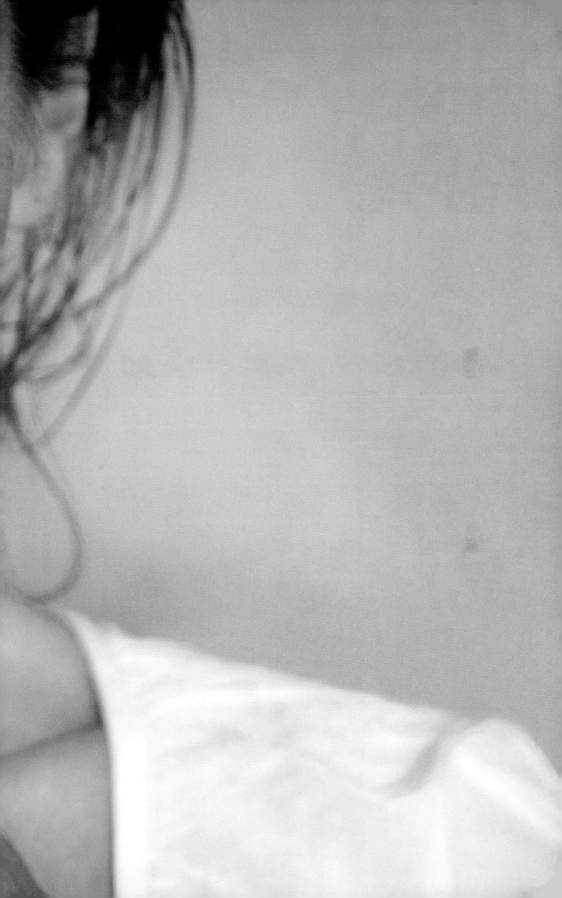

IN PRAISE OF SILENCE

Close your eyes, center yourself, and focus. If you don't hear anything, that's good. Our houses and apartments are filled with background noise from appliances, televisions, and telephones that pollute our sound environment. Silence is a precious gift. It allows us to listen to our own inner voice, revealing what we truly desire, not just what others have come to expect from us. Whenever you can, try to find a tranquil, peaceful spot for a moment of respite. Sometimes it's essential to take some uncluttered time and replenish the inner self. It makes no sense to be endlessly, needlessly, busy. Don't dread the occasional idle interlude. Relish the silence and a fleeting moment of solitude—you'll feel renewed and revitalized.

THE RIGHT WAY TO CHEW

You might suppose that chewing is as innate as breathing. But just as it's important to learn the right way to breathe, it's essential to pay attention to the way you chew your food. Once again, the best advice is to take your time. Chewing properly leads to better digestion—that's my new motto. Numerous scientific studies have shown that a sense of satiation occurs about 20 minutes after beginning a meal, so it's advisable to chew thoroughly rather than gobbling down whatever's set before you. Taking the time to chew properly aids in the absorption of glucose and speeds up the metabolization of lipids. By chewing more thoroughly, we end up eating less and eliminating more. Some nutritionists believe that eating meals more slowly can assist weight loss, and they recommend tougher foods rather than soft ones. If you're tempted to snack, I suggest you eat a few almonds, which are rich in minerals, monounsaturated fatty acids, and vegetable proteins. I always carry a packet of nuts in my handbag—they're better for you and much more natural than a pack of chewing gum!

SELF-MASSAGING THE ABDOMEN

In addition to eating slowly, you can invigorate your spleen by self-massaging your abdomen. Before going to sleep, rub your abdomen 80 times in each direction. The warmth of your hands will produce a gentle sensation of well-being for both the spleen and stomach.

"The greatest revelation is silence."

LAO-TZU

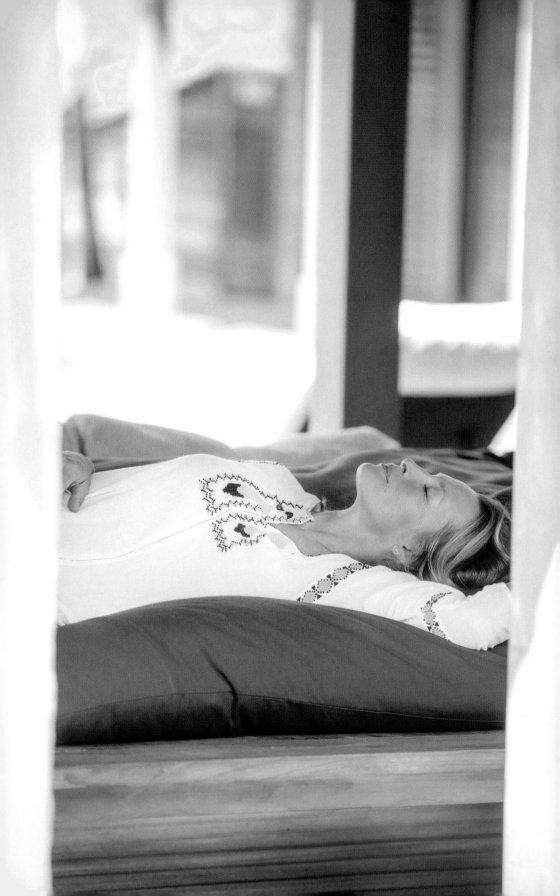

ADVICE FROM A NATUROPATHIC SPECIALIST
FOCUS ON THE STOMACH

Summer is waning, and the heat waves are over. Autumn hasn't yet arrived: the days are still sunny with low humidity. But the leaves are turning dry and taking on their first hints of red. The hours of sunshine are shorter now, giving way to the early days of Indian summer.

Our bodies often experience fatigue during heat waves. Summer meals are not all that wholesome (ice cream, charcuterie, take-out treats), and we may overindulge in alcoholic beverages some evenings. All these problems are compounded by the bad habit of drinking orange juice at breakfast and tomato juice before meals. These drinks prevent proper digestion of the enzyme amylase in the mouth-esophagus-stomach system.

Summer often ends with a case of gastro-enteritis and recurrent digestive problems in the stomach (flatulence, slow digestion, postprandial drowsiness, etc.).

Restoring health to the stomach and pancreas
→ For three nights in a row, eat nothing but a freshly prepared puree of fresh vegetables and potatoes. Don't keep any leftovers for the next day. This simple cure will give your stomach a rest.
→ Drink this special infusion 15 minutes before lunch and dinner: mix 2 pinches of calamas root (*Acorus calamus*) + a crushed star anise flower in 2 glasses of mineral water (I like Mont Roucous or Montcalm water). Look for a natural mineral water with a very low mineral and low sodium content, such as those recommended for babies. Simmer over low heat for 5 minutes. Turn off the heat and add a few peppermint leaves, fresh if possible. Steep for 10 minutes. Drink this unsweetened tisane for several days to help your stomach function effectively.
→ Follow the general advice (p. 14).

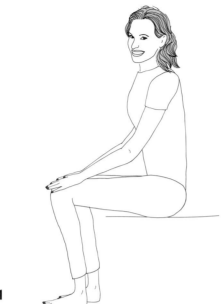

1

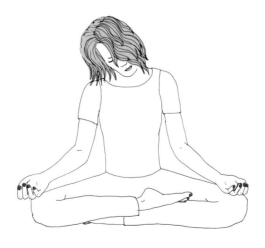

2

EXERCISES FOR INDIAN SUMMER
SEATED MEDITATION

→ Sit comfortably in a chair **(1)** or on a zafu (meditation pillow), keeping your back very straight, with your feet flat on the floor or with your legs in the lotus position (cross-legged).

→ Relax and drop your shoulders as low as possible. Rest your hands on your thighs and close your eyes. Take a few moments to relax the back of your neck by making small, slow circling movements of your head and shoulders **(2)**. Make sure you're not creating any tautness—you want just the opposite, to gently relax any areas of stiffness.

→ Now direct your attention to your breathing; take note of your inhalations and exhalations. As you breathe in, feel the air in the pelvic area, slightly contract your perineum, and stretch your body as you breathe in; then relax your body as you exhale. You can actually help the passage of air with your body's movements. Your back and neck are relaxed before inhaling, then stretched upward as far as possible at the end of the inhalation. Gradually relax your chest and perineum throughout the entire exhalation, like a deflating balloon.

→ If a thought crosses your mind, let it pass like a cloud and return to focusing on your breathing and the air that you're inhaling and exhaling. Think about its temperature and concentrate on the sensations your body is experiencing in the moment.

→ Pay attention to your breathing for 3 to 5 minutes and gradually, on your own terms and at your own pace, you'll progress to meditations of 20 to 30 minutes, enhancing the well-being of both mind and body. Think of meditation as an experience, not as a test.

THE + The perineum is active on a daily basis. This muscle is called upon every time there's abdominal pressure during breathing and the use of the abdominal muscles. It plays an essential role in continence, childbirth, sexual activity, and overall body energy. It is therefore vital for both men and women to care for their bodies by strengthening the muscle tone of this area. Begin by mentally locating this muscle and practice muscle contractions on a daily basis, while brushing your teeth, for example, or while waiting in line, but especially when you're engaged in a session of abdominal exercises!

MOUTH AND LIP CARE TIPS

The lip contours

Some people will tell you to draw a dark line above and below the contours of your lips to create an impression of fullness. This look is dated and the result is generally counterproductive. If you want to make your lips look fuller, nothing works better than a pale colored lipstick to give an impression of volume.

Lip peels

The lips can get dry when the first cold snap arrives, or if you smoke. I recommend a mild weekly lip peeling with a facial exfoliant to get rid of dead skin, then moisturize your lips with a chapstick.
My personal favorite is Mixa balm. I've always got one at the bottom of my handbag. Or try Christophe Robin's legendary Intense Regenerating balm (available on christophe-robin.com/en)—it's good for everything. Carmex Original Stick is also effective.

Mouth exercises

To keep your mouth area firm and well toned, there's nothing more effective than this little gymnastic exercise. Every morning, whether snugly tucked in under your quilt or standing in front of the bathroom mirror, make alternate "Ahhh" and "Eeee" sounds—a dozen of each—and finish up with a big wide smile. Nothing beats this routine if you want to start the day on an energetic note.

THE RIGHT TOOTHPASTE

The presence of sodium fluoride in our water, foodstuffs, and many other products is increasingly being called into question. So choose an organic toothpaste that's free of fluoride, and once a week brush your teeth using a teaspoon of baking soda mixed with a few drops of essential tea tree oil. And to make sure you have fresh-smelling breath, rinse your mouth with a few drops of peppermint oil.

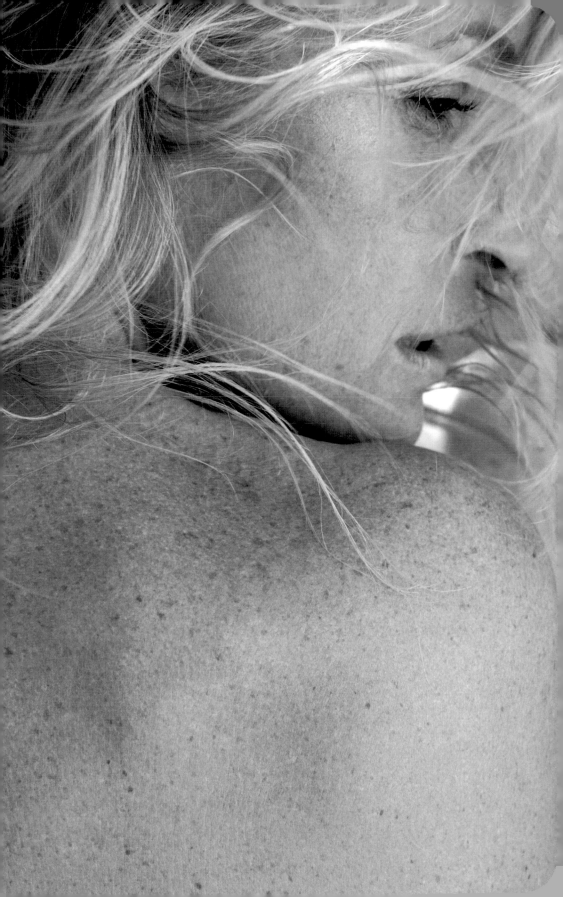

My seasonal market basket

Fruits
Apples
Blackberries
Blueberries
Figs
Grapes
Melons
Mirabelle plums
Nectarines
Peaches
Pears
Raspberries

...

Vegetables
Artichokes
Beets
Bell peppers
Broccoli
Carrots
Cauliflowers
Celery
Cucumbers
Eggplants
Fennel
Green beans
Leeks
Lettuces
Radishes
Spinach
Zucchini

...

FENNEL

Very popular in southern Europe, especially in Italy, fennel was used by the Romans against scorpion stings and by the Chinese to treat snakebites. You'll find fennel bulbs in the market from the beginning of June until the beginning of winter (in the northern hemisphere).

With its many valuable nutritional properties, fennel has a positive effect on bone health, as well as on hypertension. It is known as a remedy for coughs and colds. Rich in antioxidants, particularly flavonoids, it also contains polyacetylenes, which have antibacterial and anti-inflammatory effects. It's a good source of vitamin C, too. Relished for its licorice flavor, fennel is delicious raw or cooked, in both savory and sweet dishes. You can enjoy it in a salad or a braised dish, compote, or soup—there's no end of recipe possibilities. When I want to surprise my guests, I serve fennel in a fruit salad that includes apples, oranges, and apricots.

My Fruit Salad with Fennel

1 fennel bulb
2 oranges
3 apples
4 mirabelle plums

Wash the fennel bulb and the fruits. Remove the peel from the oranges. Cut all the ingredients into small pieces and mix together in a bowl.

Younger-by-a-Decade Rejuvenating Smoothie

Serves 2

Ingredients
1 cup (225 ml) coconut milk
4 oz. (125 g) pineapple,
  chopped
1 banana, peeled and
  chopped
1 tablespoon coconut oil
½ teaspoon ground turmeric
½ teaspoon ground
  cinnamon
½ teaspoon ground ginger
1 teaspoon chia seeds
1 teaspoon maca powder

To prepare the smoothie
This is a very simple anti-aging recipe. Put all the ingredients in a blender and blend until smooth. Pour into tall glasses and enjoy!

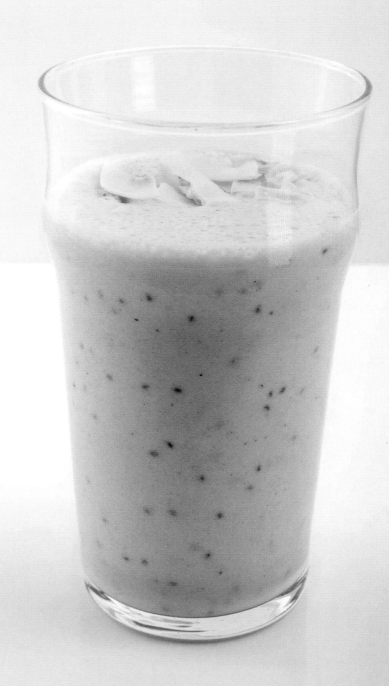

Sexy Bowl

<u>Serves 2</u>

Ingredients
1 medium sweet potato

For the sauce
⅓ cup (80 ml) orange juice
1 teaspoon white miso
1 teaspoon maca powder
1 teaspoon pumpkin seed oil
1 teaspoon finely grated
  orange zest

For the salad
1 large zucchini, cut into
  ½ in. (1 cm) rounds
2 tablespoons coconut oil
½ avocado, peeled, pitted,
  and chopped
3 oz. (60 g) white cabbage,
  shredded
1 sheet of nori, cut into fine
  strips
A few radish sprouts
A few pumpkin seeds

To cook the sweet potato
Preheat the oven to 400°F (200°C/Gas Mark 6). Scrub the sweet potato and prick it with a fork. Cook on the middle shelf of the oven for 50 minutes, until it is tender.

To prepare the sauce
While the sweet potato bakes, put all the sauce ingredients into a blender and blend until smooth and creamy. Pour the sauce into a bowl and set aside.

Sauté the zucchini rounds in a little coconut oil over medium heat until they are just golden. Remove the zucchini from the pan and divide between two serving plates.

Remove the sweet potato from the oven, cut in half, and strip off the skin. Arrange one half on each plate.

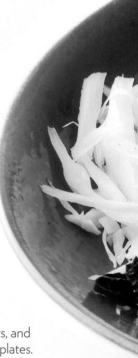

Divide the avocado, white cabbage, nori strips, radish sprouts, and pumpkin seeds between the two plates.

Serve with the sauce. Eat while the sweet potato and zucchini are still warm.

Sexy Secret
This salad qualifies as sexy because its ingredients include maca powder, the Peruvian answer to ginseng. It stimulates the production of sex hormones and minimizes the symptoms of menopause.

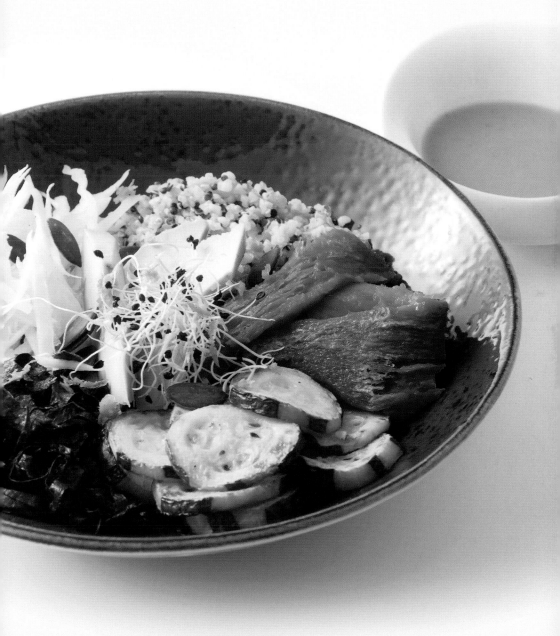

Eggplant with Yogurt

Serves 4

Ingredients
For the yogurt sauce
1 small cucumber
¾ cup (200 ml) sheep milk
   yogurt
1 teaspoon toasted sesame
   seeds
Finely grated zest of 1 lemon
1 tablespoon chopped fresh
   mint leaves
Salt and pepper

For the salad
2 eggplants
1 garlic clove, peeled and
   chopped
1 shallot, peeled and
   chopped
6 tablespoons organic olive
   oil
½ cup (100 ml) soy sauce
3 tablespoons lemon juice
1 package mixed green salad
   leaves

To prepare the sauce
Peel the cucumber, remove the seeds, and cut into small pieces. In a bowl, combine the cucumber, yogurt, toasted sesame seeds, the lemon zest, and the fresh mint. Season to taste.

To prepare the salad
Wash and peel the eggplants and cut into ¾ in. (2 cm) pieces. Sauté the garlic and shallots in the olive oil and then add the eggplant pieces and soy sauce. Cook over low heat for about 20 minutes, stirring often. When done, add the lemon juice. Combine the salad leaves and eggplant before adding the yogurt sauce.

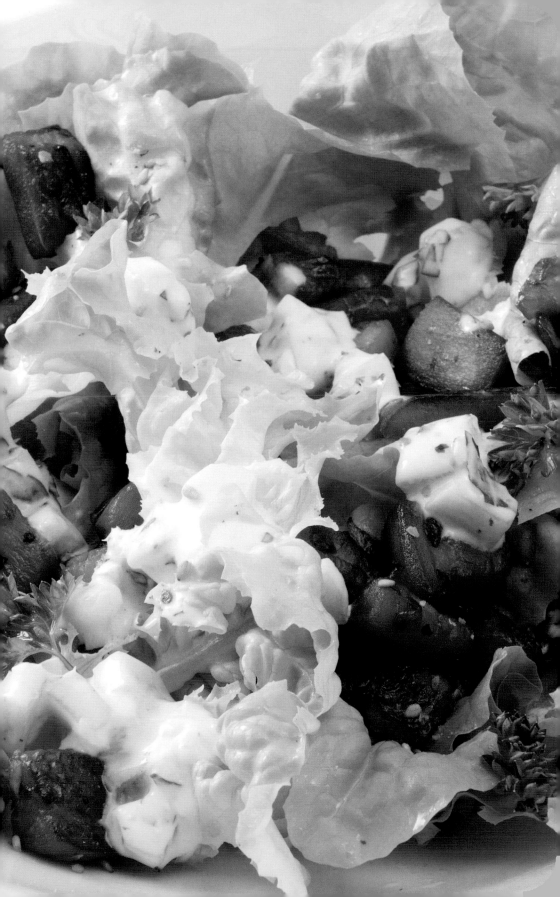

Toffuccino

Serves 6

Ingredients
1 small cup of single espresso
10 oz. (300 g) dark
   chocolate, chopped,
   plus extra grated
   chocolate for sprinkling
7 oz. (200 g) silken tofu
2 egg whites
1 pinch of salt
1 ½ tablespoons coconut
   flower sugar

To prepare the toffuccino
Pour the espresso into the top of a double boiler or bain-marie. Add the chopped dark chocolate and let it melt completely. Stir the mixture with a spatula until smooth and then pour it into a blender.

Thoroughly drain the silken tofu, add it to the chocolate, and mix in before blending everything together.

Beat the two egg whites with a pinch of salt until peaks form. Whisking constantly, add the coconut flower sugar. Fold the beaten egg whites and chocolate mixture together until combined—do this carefully so you don't knock the air out of the whites and they lose their volume. Refrigerate for about 4 hours.

Before serving, sprinkle each serving with grated dark chocolate.

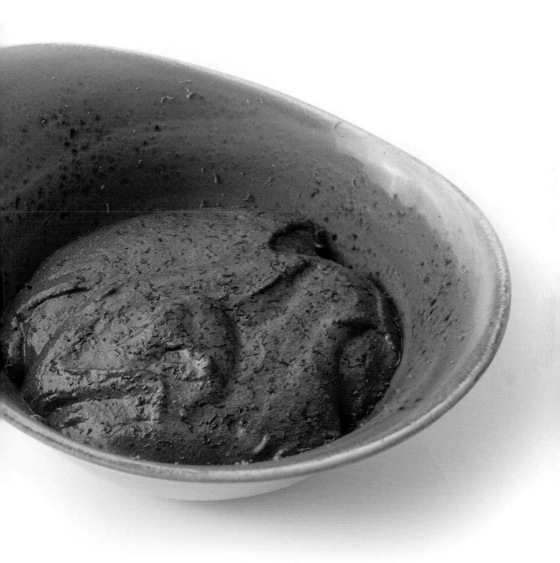

Recipe from Alain Pegouret
Le Laurent restaurant, Paris
Roasted Cod with Black Olives, Mi-Cuit Tomatoes, Basil, and Eggplant Caviar

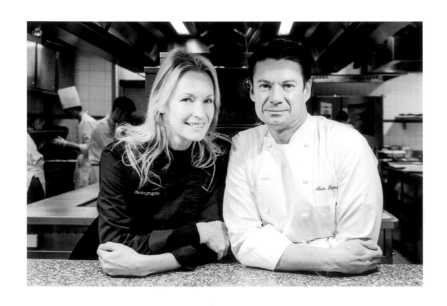

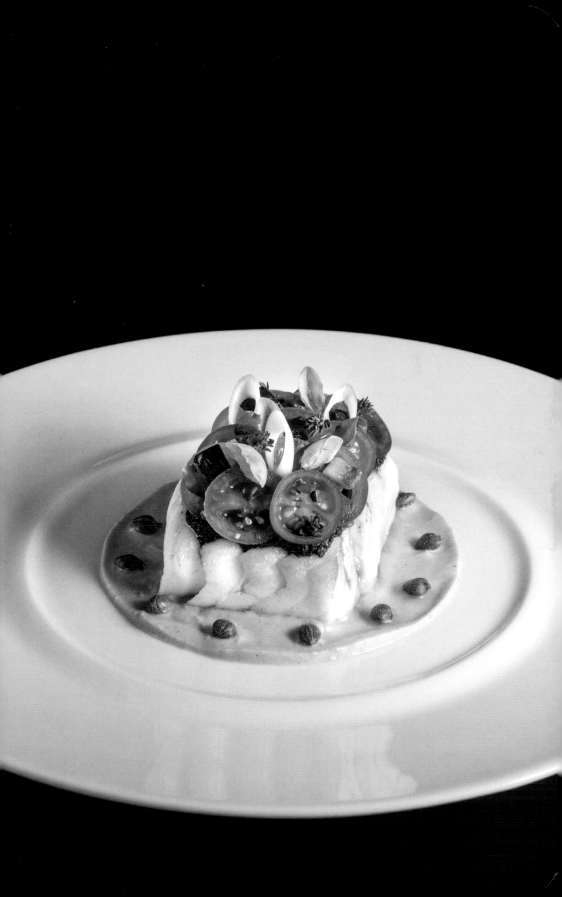

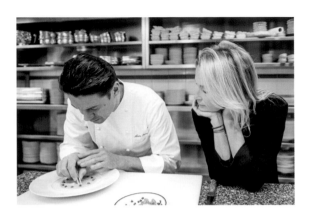
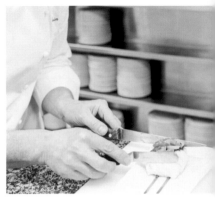

Serves 4

Ingredients
1 cod fillet, weighing
    4 lb. 8 oz. (2 kg), skin
    and bones removed

For the marinade
1 ¼ cups (300 g) kosher salt
1 cup (200 g) granulated
    sugar
2 teaspoons freshly ground
    pepper
3 juniper berries, crushed
Olive oil

For the eggplant caviar
5 eggplants
Kosher salt
½ cup (100 ml) olive oil
2 teaspoons basil-flavored
    olive oil
6 tablespoons finely sliced
    scallions
1 tablespoon finely chopped
    garlic
2 tablespoons lemon juice
2 teaspoons fine salt
1 pinch of freshly ground
    pepper

1 pinch of ground cumin
2 ½ tablespoons mayonnaise

For the garnish
8 cocktail tomatoes,
    pineapple variety
8 cocktail tomatoes, black
    Crimean variety
8 red cocktail tomatoes
2 tablespoons black olive
    tapenade
1 scallion, finely sliced
    on the diagonal
20 leaves of basil cress
10 pitted black olives, halved
20 garlic flower petals
1 pinch of garlic scapes
    powder
Thyme flowers
40 small capers

For the seasonings
Fine salt and freshly ground
    pepper
Crushed black pepper
Olive oil
Sherry vinegar

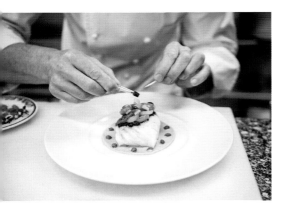

Blend the eggplant pulp with the other caviar ingredients in a food processor. Strain the puree through a sieve lined with cheesecloth. Set aside.

To prepare the garnish
Wash all the tomatoes and slice into very thin rounds, ⅛ in. (3 mm) thick.

To cook the cod and finish
Reheat the oven to 350°F (180°C/Gas Mark 4). Sauté the pieces of cod in olive oil in a nonstick skillet until three-quarters cooked. Remove from the pan and spread them with the black olive tapenade. Arrange rounds of tomato on top, alternating the different varieties.

Sprinkle the tomatoes with a fine drizzle of olive oil, season with kosher salt and freshly ground pepper, and finish cooking in the oven.

Spread a 4 in. (10 cm) circle of eggplant caviar, 1 ¼ in. (3 cm) thick, on four serving plates. Position the cod fillets in the center. Arrange the sliced scallion, basil cress, black olives, garlic petals, garlic scapes powder, and thyme flowers attractively on top of the tomatoes. Season with a few drops of sherry vinegar and finish by placing the capers on the eggplant caviar and adding a few drops of olive oil.

To marinate the cod
For the marinade, mix the salt and sugar together with the freshly ground pepper and juniper berries. Put half of this mixture in a baking dish, place the cod fillet on top, and cover with the rest of the mixture. Marinate for 45 minutes.

At the end of this time, rinse the cod fillet in cold water, dry it carefully with paper towel. Cover the cod with olive oil and leave for 6 hours. Drain the cod, divide into four identical size portions, and set aside in the refrigerator.

To prepare the eggplant caviar
Preheat the oven to 350°F (180°C/Gas Mark 4). Prick the eggplants with a fork. Spread a 1 ¼ in. (3 cm) layer of kosher salt on a baking sheet. Arrange the eggplants on top, side by side, and bake in the oven for 45 minutes until tender.

When the eggplants are ready, remove them from the oven and let cool for 15 minutes. Cut the eggplants in half lengthwise and scoop out the pulp with a large spoon.

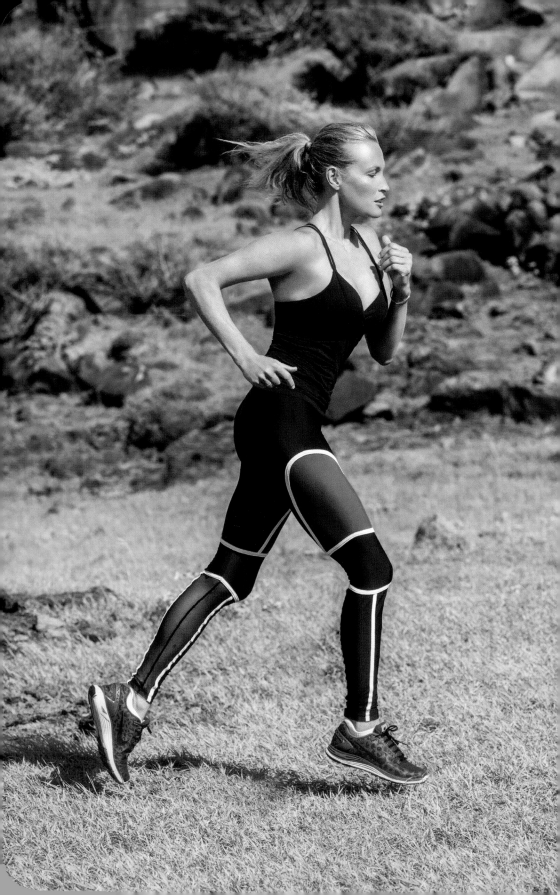

Autumn

"Autumn: the time for man and nature to follow the path together, both their lifespans drawing to a close."

Autumn is a windy, stormy season. When the first red leaves appear on the trees and the days grow shorter, chills and coughs come back in force.

Traditional Chinese medicine tells us that autumn is the time to pay special attention to the lungs. Healthy breathing provides the body with its oxygen supply, the source of vitality and youth. In combination with hydrogen, oxygen assures the healthy functioning of all our cells. You should pay attention to repeated sneezes, a stuffy nose, or a sensation of congestion in the sinuses. These symptoms indicate that there is blockage in the lungs. Ailments such as laryngitis or sore throat demonstrate vulnerability. The condition of your skin is also a reliable indicator. Obstructed pores, for example, indicate that respiratory function is affected, and dry skin is a sign that there is a problem with the body's fluid distribution system.

Teach yourself how to breathe properly. We all think we know how to do this, but breathing correctly is a priority in controlling stress and eliminating toxins. Along with these daily exercises, I recommend a nice infusion of thyme leaves, which have antiseptic properties.

THE RIGHT WAY TO BREATHE

Proper breathing sends a vital signal to the reptilian part of the brain that we are in control of a situation. Through practicing yoga and Pilates, I've been able to master several breathing techniques that help you to feel better.

A little exercise for cardiac function

This is an exercise that I often practice as it's simple, effective, and easy to remember:
→ 3 times a day;
→ 6 breaths per minute;
→ for 5 minutes.

Breathing through alternate nostrils

Those who practice Hatha yoga will be familiar with this exercise under its Indian name of *anulom ailom pranayama*. It's said to be an outstanding antidote to stress and anxiety.
→ Begin by closing your eyes. Close your right nostril with your right thumb. Breathe in deeply through your left nostril until your lungs are filled with air.
→ Hold your breath, closing the open nostril with your right ring finger. Then, exhale slowly through your right nostril.
→ Breathe in through your right nostril. Close your right nostril, hold your breath, and open the left nostril. Exhale through the left nostril, and so on.

To maximize the efficacy of this exercise, it's recommended that you do at least 5 repetitions. Finish by breathing in and exhaling deeply.

"The more you have, the more you are occupied. The less you have, the more free you are."

MOTHER TERESA

THINK ABOUT YOURSELF

Autumn marks the end of summer vacation, the resumption of work, the start of the school year, and all the stress that goes along with these changes. It is absolutely essential not to lose your sense of self. Don't become overwhelmed by onrushing events. It's vitally important to dedicate a few minutes or an hour each day to your own well-being.

LEARNING HOW TO SAY NO TO YOURSELF

We often hear how important it is to say no to others, or reject certain situations or obligations. But the one person we rarely say no to is our own self. No, I'm not going to deal with those bills now. No, I'm not going to wash the dishes right away. Right now, I'm going to take a moment to enjoy myself. I'm going to watch a good film, have coffee with a friend, play a sport I love. I'll make myself the priority!

Unless you're Superwoman, it's impossible for you to have everything perfect and under control all the time. Learning how to postpone some chores is an essential first step in discovering how to unwind.

AN UNWINDING EXERCISE

This exercise, inspired by Ayurvedic practices, should be done whenever you need to feel revitalized.

Sit down in a chair. Raise your arms, fists closed, toward the sky, breathing in through the nose and contracting the upper body. Release with a swift movement, opening your hands toward the ground as if flinging out your fingers, exhaling loudly through the mouth and relaxing the body completely. Repeat 10 times to feel completely reenergized.

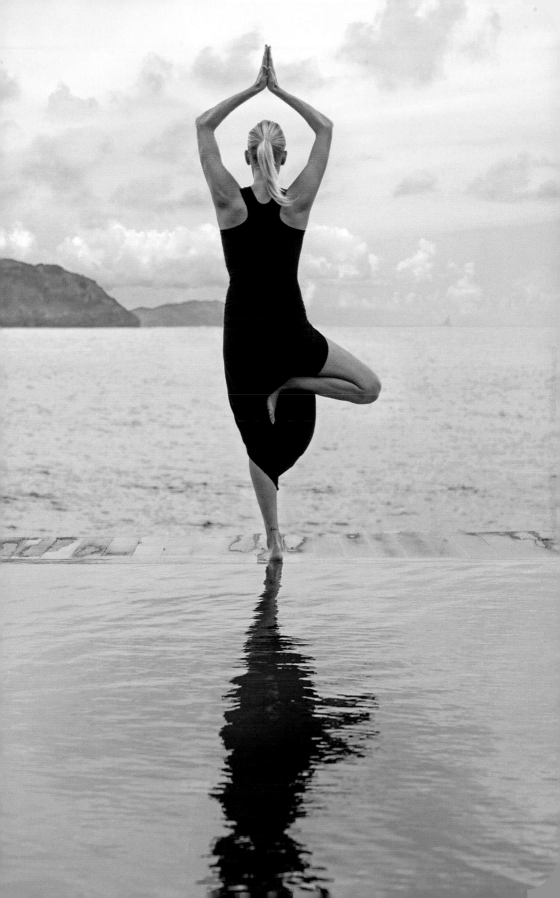

ADVICE FROM A NATUROPATHIC SPECIALIST
FOCUS ON THE LUNGS

Autumn brings rain, fog, and abrupt drops in temperature, all of which depress the bronchial and pulmonary immune systems. A variety of infections can occur with little forewarning.

Everyone is familiar with the negative impact of tobacco and alcohol on the immune system, but there are three nutritional factors that seriously compromise immunity:
→ snacking;
→ protein deficiency;
→ excessive consumption of high water content fruits.

And also:
→ high exposure to electromagnetic fields;
→ inadequate sleep.

So, avoid snacking. Reduce consumption of fruits that have a high water content (oranges, grapefruits, apples, pears, clementines, etc.) to 9 oz. (250 g) a day for those who are ruddy-skinned and not sensitive to cold and 2–4 oz. (50–125 g) a day for pale-skinned individuals vulnerable to chills. These fruits should be eaten only between 5:30 and 6:00 p.m. In addition, proteins (meat, seafood, fish, or eggs) must be included in the midday meal every day.

Certain plants enhance the efficiency of the immune system:
→ Echinacea, especially if it is from fresh plants. Try taking 20 drops of echinacea morning and evening, to which you should add 10 drops of wild rosebud oil. Whatever your age, these two plant essences taken together in a glass of spring water will give you protection from various winter ailments.
→ For head and neck or bronchial infections, take echinacea + wild rose morning and evening. On even-numbered days, take a copper-gold-silver supplement and on odd-numbered days a manganese-copper capsule. Continue until the symptoms are eliminated. The treatment will thus be gradually reduced.
→ Also follow the general advice (p. 14).

Ten tips for the first cold snap

Make sure your head, hands, and feet are well covered

Don't overheat your home or office

Take a vitamin C cure

Eat dried vegetables such as beans and peas

Wash your hands frequently

Scent your handkerchiefs with essential mint oil

Practice deep breathing

Drink infusions of thyme

Open the windows to let air circulate

Use light to combat feelings of depression

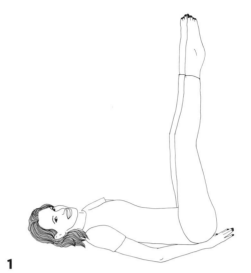

1

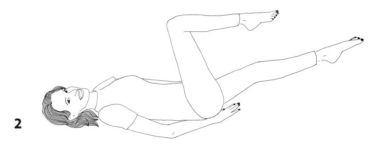

2

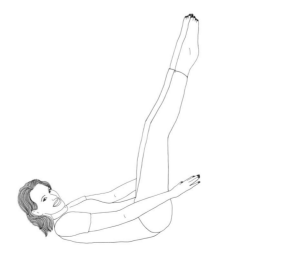

3

EXERCISES FOR AUTUMN
DANCING SCISSORS AND CORE TRAINING ON YOUR BACK

→ Stretch out on your back, with your arms at your sides and your chin tucked in. Raise your legs to a vertical position **(1)**. Use the core of your body from this point on.

→ As you inhale, lower your right leg rapidly to about 1 inch (2–3 cm) above the floor while bending the left leg **(2)**. Hold this position for 2 seconds, then sit up, breathing through your mouth, while vigorously contracting the perineum and stomach. Switch legs. Do between 15 and 20 repetitions. Your abdominal muscles will feel the burn!

→ Raise your legs to a vertical position and point your toes, then flex them in a V, with the heels and ankles together (this will make you feel the contraction of your adductor muscles more intensely). Now tighten your abdominal muscles and lower your legs to a 45 degree angle, at the same time raising your chest. Pulling on your arms, raise your shoulders from the ground with your chin tucked in, while exhaling **(3)**. When you are first starting this exercise, hold the position for at least one complete inhalation and exhalation. Work your way up to 2 to 4 in and out breaths. Always be aware of your perineum and make sure you relax and tighten your abdominal muscles.

→ Perform this sequence of two exercises 3 to 5 times. I guarantee you'll have rock-hard abdominal and perineal muscles!

→ If you have back pain, slide your hands underneath your buttocks and slightly bend your knees **(1)**. This movement shouldn't be painful, so adjust your body until you find a comfortable position.

→ To finish, bend both of your knees up against the abdomen, and clasp them with your arms.

THE + During these abdominal exercises, begin by contracting the perineum before the stomach. To maximize the stomach flattening effect, pull in your navel and then your lower abdomen. This will better protect your back. You'll also see encouraging results more rapidly.

HAND AND FOOT CARE TIPS

The right length

Perfectly manicured hands and feet are synonymous with good grooming. Whether you care for them at home or in a beauty salon, nails should be cut short. In my opinion, nails that are too long add several years to your age. For the normal requirements of daily life, I think this look is more contemporary, practical, and healthy.

The best nail polish

When deciding on nail polish, I generally choose a colorless base for the hands and a colored polish for my feet. I love dark colors like burgundy or navy blue on my toes. I'm especially fond of the Kure Bazaar line, whose high-style colors are all natural and based on a blend of wood pulp, cotton, corn, potatoes, and wheat. Be aware that if you use dark polish too frequently, the nails have a tendency to yellow, and small spots can appear. If this happens, my little secret remedy is to remove all the polish. Then use a Q-Tip to apply essential tea tree oil until the nails recover their natural appearance.

For lovely hands

Exposed to the damaging effects of cold, heat, water, dishwashing, and cooking, hands are particularly sensitive, and it's important to take proper care of them. I recommend using protective cooking gloves as often as possible. If they're very thin, you won't lose any sensation in your fingers while you cook.

I have two particular favorites for organic moisturizing: Mains de Reine with organic French beeswax from Folies Royales and Miel Suprême, beauty care for the hands and nails with organic linden flower honey by Sanoflore. Burt's Bees Beeswax and Banana Hand Creme or Body Shop Honeymania Hand Cream also work wonders. Thank you, busy bees!

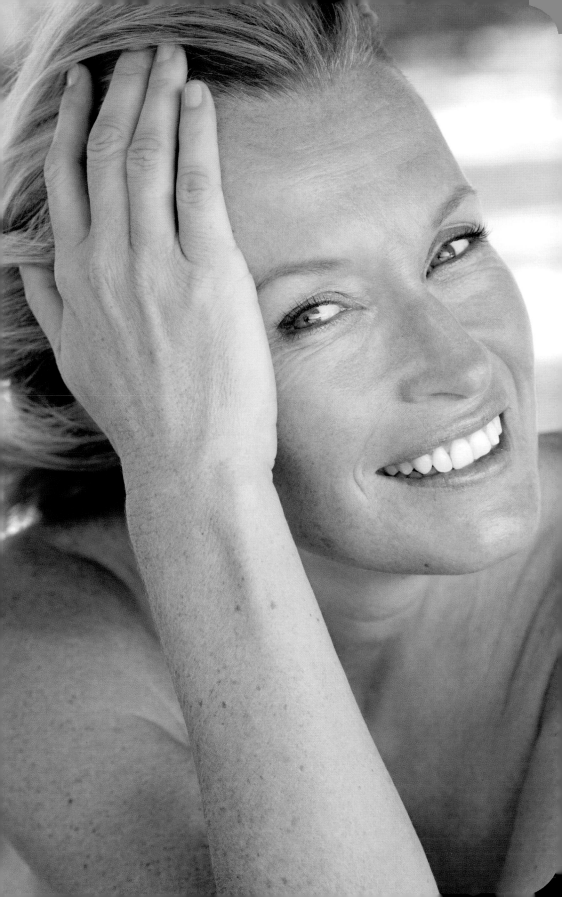

My seasonal market basket

Fruits
Apples
Chestnuts
Figs
Grapes
Pears
Plums
Quince
Raspberries
...

Vegetables
Artichokes
Beets
Broccoli
Brussels sprouts
Cabbages
Carrots
Cauliflowers
Celery
Fennel
Green beans
Leeks
Pumpkins
Radishes
Spinach
Turnips
Zucchini

...

QUINCE

Originally from Iran, quince ripens in autumn. Today the fruit is mostly used to make jellies or preserves, but the Romans used quince's essential oils to make perfumes. In eastern Europe, quince is generally treated as a vegetable. It's the main ingredient of a traditional winter soup.

Quince is rich in pectin, which helps jams and fruit preserves to gel, and it also has antioxidant properties. The fruit is always eaten cooked and unfortunately loses its vitamin C in the process. Low in sugar and calories, quince is a good source of copper and nutritional fiber. Quince can be substituted for apricots in tagine recipes. You can also combine quince with chestnuts or apples in fruit compotes.

My Quince Compote

2 small quinces
3 apples
A few almonds, chopped

Wash the quinces and peel them. Remove the seeds and dice very finely. Do the same with the apples. Simmer the diced quince, adding a little water while cooking, for about 30 minutes, adding the diced apple after 10 minutes. Once the cooking is complete, add a few chopped almonds for a bit of crunchy texture.

Emma's Cake and Spiced Warm Milk for the First Cold Snap

This cake, made from fruit compote and carrots, is an original creation by my daughter Emma.

Spiced Warm Milk
Serves 1

Ingredients
1 cup (250 ml)
   vegetable milk
   (almond, soy,
   rice, oat, etc.)
1 piece of fresh ginger,
   grated
1 cinnamon stick
1 tablespoon honey

To prepare the warm milk
Warm the vegetable milk in a small pot. Add the grated ginger, the cinnamon stick, and the honey. Allow to steep for a few minutes, and drink while hot.

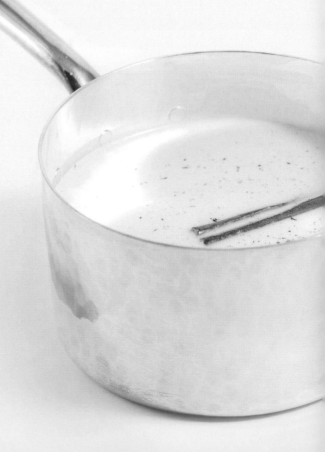

Emma's Cake
Makes 1 cake

Ingredients
1 good-sized carrot
1 banana
½ cup (100 g) organic apple
   and apricot compote
1 teaspoon cinnamon
¾ cup (165 g) coconut flower
   sugar
½ cup (125 g) organic
   vegetable margarine
1 teaspoon vanilla extract
3 tablespoons maple syrup
2 eggs
5 tablespoons organic
   almond milk
3 ½ cups (320 g) organic rice
   flour
1 teaspoon baking soda
½ teaspoon salt
1 small handful of chopped
   walnuts
Coconut oil

To prepare the cake
Peel the carrot and cut into slices. Cook in water until very tender. Preheat the oven to 320°F (160°C/ Gas Mark 3). Mash the carrot and banana. Add the organic apple and apricot compote and the cinnamon. Combine the sugar, margarine, vanilla, and maple syrup in a bowl. Add the eggs, the compote/banana/carrot mixture, and the organic almond milk.

In another bowl, combine the rice flour, baking soda, and salt. Gradually add the contents of the first bowl to the flour mixture, stirring as you go. Add the chopped walnuts.

Grease a 9 x 5 in. (23 x 13 cm) loaf pan with coconut oil and pour the batter into it. Bake for about 1 hour.

Variation
Try the same recipe replacing the compote and banana with 1 ¼ cups (300 g) of bananas.

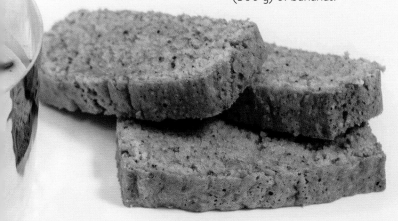

Autumn Crêpes

Serves 3

Ingredients

For the crêpes
¾ cup (90 g) spelt flour
1 pinch of salt
1 egg, beaten
1 cup (250 ml) almond
  or oat milk
1 tablespoon finely chopped
  parsley

For the chanterelles
2 tablespoons olive oil
2 shallots, peeled and finely
  chopped
3 garlic cloves, peeled and
  finely chopped
8 oz. (225 g) chanterelles,
  washed well and cut into
  thin slices
1 tablespoon finely chopped
  parsley
Salt and pepper

To prepare the crêpes

Sift the flour into a large bowl. Add the salt, egg, and half of the milk, and mix well. Gradually add the rest of the milk and the parsley.

Preheat the oven to about 250°F (130°C/Gas Mark ½). Heat and lightly oil a 10 in. (25 cm) skillet. Pour a ladle of the batter into the pan, swirling it so it spreads out evenly over the base in a nice thin crêpe. Cook the crêpe for about 30 seconds on each side until browned. Remove the crêpes from the pan as they cook and keep them warm in the oven.

To prepare the chanterelles

Reheat the same skillet over low heat. Add the olive oil and, when the pan is hot, sauté the chopped shallot and garlic. Add the chanterelles and continue to stir for 8–10 minutes or until they are tender. Season them with salt and pepper to taste.

Transfer the mushrooms to a platter and sprinkle with the parsley. Remove the crêpes from the oven and serve immediately with the chanterelles.

Variation

For a gluten-free recipe, replace the spelt flour with chestnut flour.

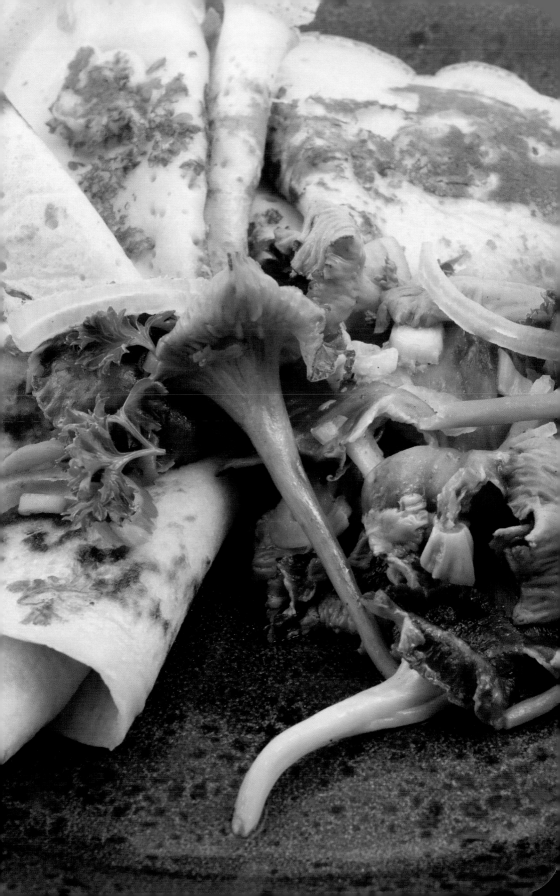

Cabbage Surprises

Serves 4

Ingredients

¼ green cabbage
4 oz. (125 g) celery root, peeled
2 carrots, peeled
1 small butternut squash, peeled and seeded
1 large shallot, peeled and finely chopped
1 garlic clove, peeled and finely chopped
1 tablespoon coconut oil
¾ cup (200 ml) vegetable bouillon
Salt and pepper

To prepare the cabbage surprises

Remove the largest cabbage leaves and blanch these in boiling water. Drain and immerse them in ice water to preserve their fresh green color. Drain again.

Cut up the remaining cabbage, celery root, carrots, and butternut squash into chunks. Sauté the chopped shallot and garlic in the coconut oil. Add the vegetables, pour the bouillon over them, and season to taste. Cook over low heat for about 25 minutes.

Preheat the oven to 325°F (160°C/Gas Mark 3). Stuff the blanched cabbage leaves with the vegetable mixture, rolling the leaves around the stuffing to make little parcels with a surprise filling. Lay the parcels side by side in a baking dish and cook in the oven for about 15 minutes.

You can accompany the cabbage parcels with a grilled chicken breast.

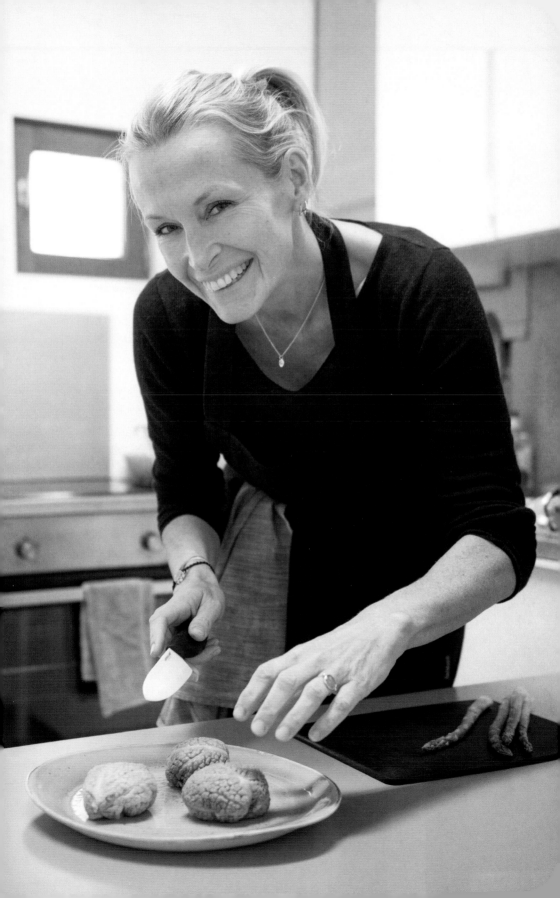

Apples Fit for a King

Serves 4

Ingredients
12 dried apricots
2 Medjool dates, pitted
4 King of the Pippens apples
    (or other variety suitable
    for baking)
A few toasted pine nuts

To prepare the dried fruit
Begin by making a dried fruit caramel,
which must be started a day in advance.

Cut the apricots into pieces, place them
in a bowl, and add the dates. Fill the bowl
with water and leave to soak in a cool
place overnight. Lift out the dried fruits
and blend them in a food processor,
adding water from the bowl gradually in
order to achieve the desired consistency,
which should resemble a thick compote.

To prepare the baked apples
Preheat the oven to 400°F (200°C/Gas
Mark 6).

Core the apples, but don't peel them.
Put the apples in a baking dish and bake
for about 30 minutes until they are nicely
browned.

Fill the center of each apple with the
dried fruit caramel and then scatter
a few toasted pine nuts on top.

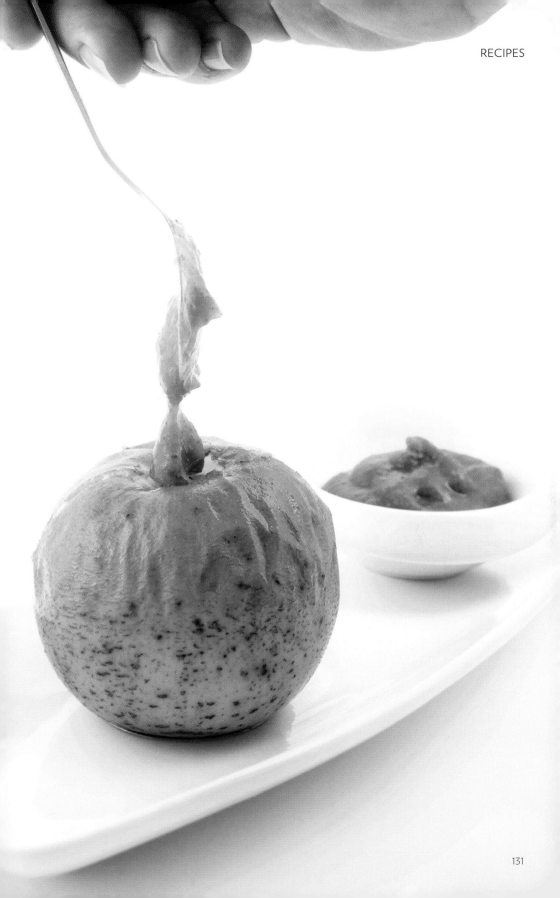

Recipe from Hélène Darroze
The Connaught hotel, London

Marinated Langoustines with a Chilled Hanoi Consommé

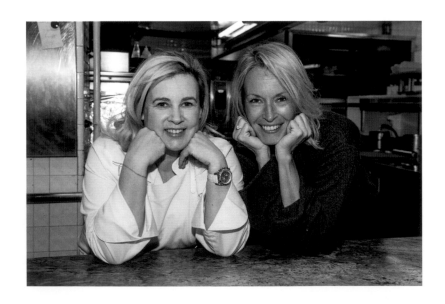

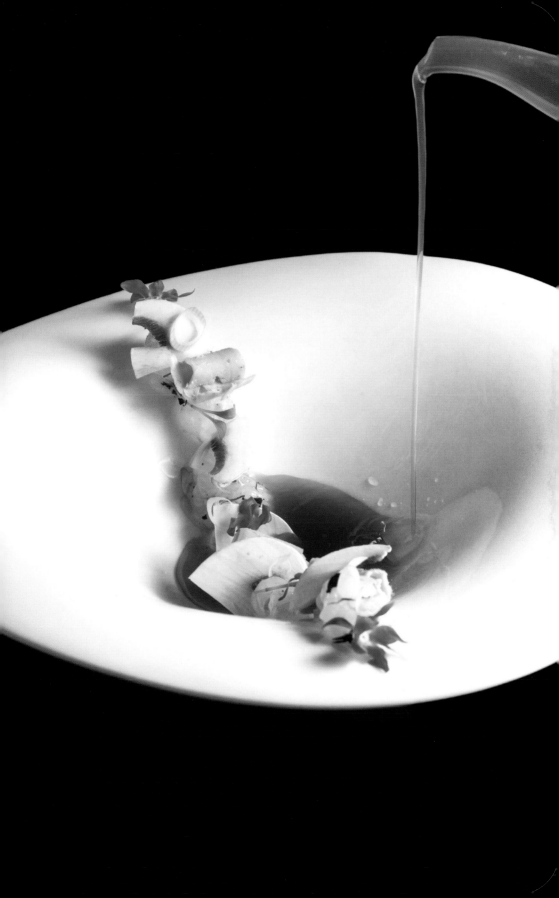

Serves 5

Ingredients
For the bouillon
4 lb. 8 oz. (2 kg)
    langoustines
5 oz. (150 g) onions
10 oz. (300 g) carrots
3 ½ oz. (100 g) fresh ginger,
    peeled and chopped
3 tablespoons coriander seeds
1 oz. (25 g) garlic cloves,
    peeled and chopped
1 star anise
1 cinnamon stick
1 teaspoon cardamom pods
1 teaspoon juniper berries
1 teaspoon black
    peppercorns
3 tablespoons nuoc-mam
    sauce
1 bunch of Vietnamese
    coriander (Vietnamese
    mint)

For the infusion
1 bunch of cilantro
1 lemon, sliced
1 bunch of fresh basil

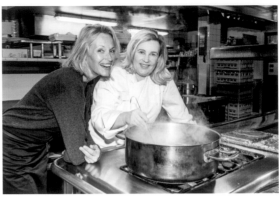

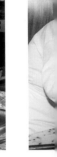

For the langoustines
Tail meat from 4 lb. 8 oz.
    (2 kg) langoustines
Lemon juice
1 bunch of cilantro
3 ½ oz. (100 g) white button mushrooms
Olive oil
½ teaspoon salt
1 pinch of ground *piment d'Espelette*
Lemon zest
2 ½ oz. (75 g) marinated foie gras, cut
    into slivers
½ oz. (10 g) cilantro micro-greens
5 borage flowers
5 violet flowers
5 mizuna flowers
Kosher salt

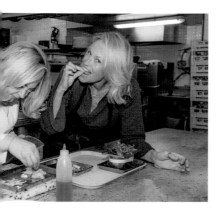
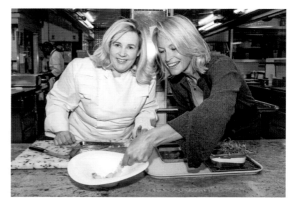

To prepare the bouillon

Carefully peel the langoustines, retaining their shells. Put the tail meat on a plate lined with paper towel and keep chilled.

Preheat the oven to 225°F (110°C/Gas Mark ¼). Dry the langoustine shells in the oven for 7 hours. Transfer the dried shells to a large soup pot and add enough water to cover them. Bring to a boil and cook for 40 minutes, skimming often.

Top up with cold water and add all the rest of the ingredients. Let simmer for about 5 hours.

Add the cilantro, lemon, and fresh basil and let infuse for 40 minutes. Strain through a fine-mesh sieve, cool, and keep chilled.

To prepare the langoustines

Bring a large pot of salted water with a little lemon juice added to it to a steady boil, submerge the langoustine tails, and cook for 1 minute. Drain and let cool.

Wash and finely chop the cilantro and the mushrooms.

Cut the langoustine tails into small pieces and set aside on a plate. Add the chopped cilantro and mushrooms.

Season with 2 tablespoons of olive oil, the salt, and *piment d'Espelette*. Sprinkle with a dash of lemon juice and grate a bit of lemon zest on top.

To serve

Arrange the langoustines attractively in soup dishes. Add a few slivers of marinated foie gras and finish by garnishing with the cilantro micro-greens, a dash of olive oil, the borage, violet and mizuna flowers, and a sprinkle of kosher salt. Just before serving, pour the chilled Hanoi consommé into each bowl.

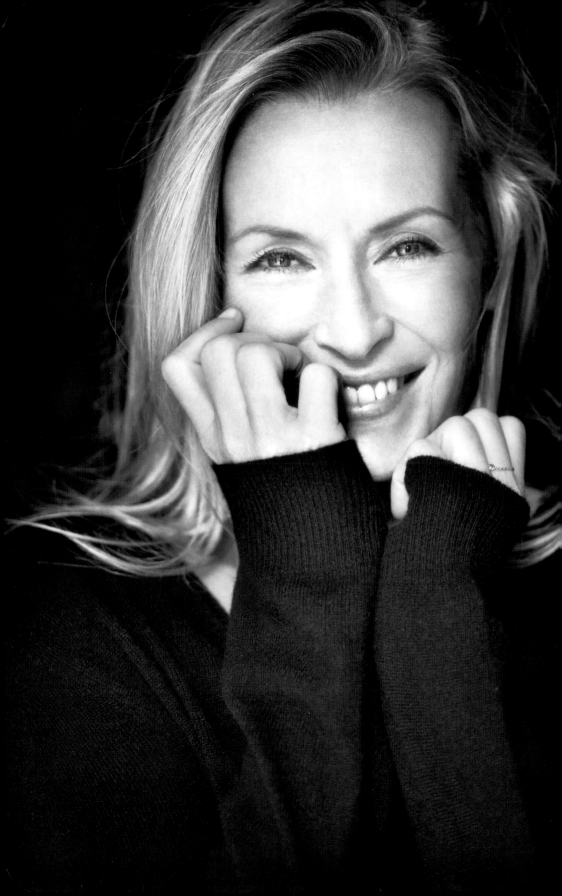

Winter

"Winter: the time when we count time."

W inter is a season of flux. When the first chilly mornings arrive and the nights grow longer than the days, we have a tendency to turn inward and hibernate. But this season can be an opportunity to recharge our batteries and renew our inner selves.

Chinese medicine teaches us that this is the season to pay particular attention to our kidneys, whose good health is synonymous with youthfulness and longevity. Since the body is made up of over 70 percent water, dehydration has an aging effect, while hydration promotes a healthy life.

Our hair reflects our general state of health. Soft, glossy tresses indicate a good level of hydration, while dry, broken, or prematurely gray hair is often a sign of mineral deficiencies. It's important to learn how to keep appropriately hydrated, but you should also understand how to avoid the causes of dry skin, wrinkles, joint problems, and pain.

So, go with the flow!

HOW TO AVOID DEHYDRATION

Here is a list of foods, products, and situations to avoid:
→ overly spicy or salty food
→ excessive consumption of meat or fatty foods
→ coffee, alcohol, and cigarettes
→ sleepless nights
→ going to bed too late
→ postprandial naps
→ heavy dinners
→ excessive sun exposure
→ excessive sexual activity
→ inactivity

HOW TO STAY WELL HYDRATED

Here is a list of recommended foods and activities:
→ nuts
→ vegetable proteins
→ green vegetables
→ seasonal fruits
→ soups
→ sparkling water rich in sodium and phosphorus
→ mineral water in glass bottles
→ eating meals at regular times
→ sleep and relaxation
→ deep breathing
→ thalassotherapy
→ postprandial strolls

A LITTLE TEST

Tug lightly at the skin on the back of your hand and immediately let it go. If your skin is well hydrated, it will spring back like an elastic band. If your skin is dehydrated, it will stay wrinkled for a moment.

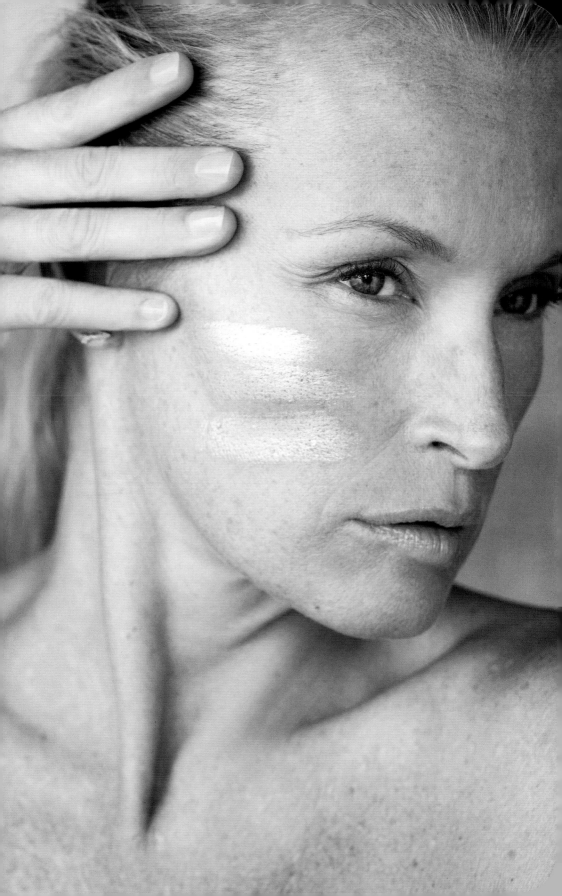

MY CREATIVE VISION OF A BETTER LIFE

Suppose we took advantage of long winter evenings to visualize our most deeply desired goals, dreams, and longings. It's a simple idea; all you do is identify these wishes as clearly as you can and embrace the belief that we have power over our own lives. The subconscious will direct you toward the actions that will transform your aspirations into reality.

And here's some good news—this exercise in creative visualization costs no more than the price of paper, scissors, and glue. Envisioning success requires no investment whatsoever, except some time and reflection. It's best to do this on your own, or with close friends, having first collected together old newspapers and magazines.

To begin, decide how you will undertake the project:
→ Use an entire wall in your home?
→ A large white or colored piece of cardboard?
→ A little compartmented file that you can easily carry with you?

All you have to do is post drawings, photos, and quotations that inspire you. What makes you dream? Write down words that motivate you. Try to always formulate your thoughts positively, picturing yourself surrounded by abundance rather than deprivation.

The objective is to reflect sincerely and profoundly on your deepest longings, whether in private or professional spheres, in family life, romance, or any other area of your life that is important to you.

It's up to you to take charge of your life!

STAY NICE AND WARM

Did you know that the Chinese and Japanese cover the kidneys with a flannel belt to keep them nice and warm in winter? In the Far East, internal warmth is synonymous with youth and vitality.

"EVERYTHING IN YOUR ENTIRE LIFE REFLECTS THE CHOICES YOU HAVE MADE. IF YOU WISH FOR A DIFFERENT RESULT, MAKE A DIFFERENT CHOICE."

ADVICE FROM A NATUROPATHIC SPECIALIST
FOCUS ON THE KIDNEYS

Winter, humidity, cold (especially around the feet), and a sedentary lifestyle all have very harmful effects on the kidneys. If you have bags under your eyes, mild swelling in your ankles, or foamy urine, these are indications of renal stress.

To protect and strengthen the kidneys, avoid excessive sodium (in prepared foods, canned goods, preserved meats) and excessive protein consumption.

Consider the impact of a starter of cured meats + a main course of a roast or steak + cheese + dessert, prepared with milk and eggs, eaten both at lunch and dinner. That's ten helpings of protein a day! And that kind of consumption is not uncommon. Excessive protein gradually destroys kidney function and, like all forms of overeating, can lead to various forms of cancer and a shorter life span.

Although inadequate amounts of protein are detrimental to the immune system, excessive consumption is harmful to kidney function. It's all a matter of moderation.

For balanced nutrition, follow the general advice (p. 14) and the alternating treatment described below for one or two months:

→ For the first two weeks of the month, drink an unsweetened tisane of cherry stems 15 minutes before the midday and evening meal. To prepare this, place a handful of cherry stems in 1 pint of spring water. Bring to a boil for 3 minutes over low heat and steep for 10 minutes. Strain and drink the tisane in two or three servings, 15 minutes before meals.

→ In the second half of the month, make a different unsweetened tea from corn silk, to be drunk 15 minutes before the morning and evening meals. To prepare, put a handful of corn silk in 1 pint of spring water. Bring to a boil for 3 minutes over low heat and steep for 10 minutes. Strain, and drink in two or three servings before meals.

→ If it's not possible for you to prepare these tisanes, you can instead drink a glass of spring water every three days, 15 minutes before the evening meal, with a capsule of linden sapwood extract.

WHOLEGRAIN SESAME

Go ahead and enjoy magical wholegrain sesame seeds. Black, brown, or creamy white, they are absolutely delicious. You can use them in a decoction with cinnamon or ginger (¾ oz./20 g per 2 cups/500 ml of water, steeped for about 30 minutes) or sprinkled over a salad. Sesame is naturally rich in minerals and trace elements (calcium, phosphorus, potassium, and magnesium), fatty acids, and proteins, and it's a great aid in supporting kidney health.

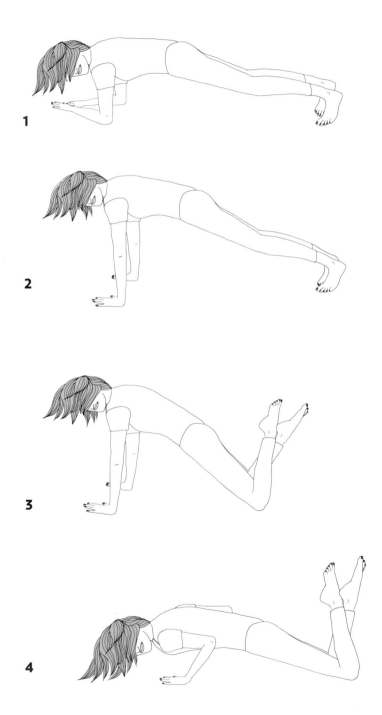

1

2

3

4

EXERCISES FOR WINTER
THE BOARD

➜ Position yourself on all fours, supported by your forearms, with elbows beneath your shoulders. Extend your legs alternately, resting on your forearms and toes. Your body should be straight, with your neck and head extending the line of your back and legs **(1)**. Your neck should be stretched out, with your eyes looking down, and your heels should be pushed back.

➜ Activate the core of your body, relaxing and contracting your perineal and stomach muscles. Maintain this position for 5 to 10 deep breaths (30 to 60 seconds).

➜ Move from supporting yourself on your forearms to supporting yourself on arms stretched straight with elbows locked **(2)**, one arm at a time and starting with your right arm, to raise your chest away from the floor. Then immediately lower yourself onto your elbows, one arm at a time, beginning with your right arm.

➜ Repeat 5 times on this side (beginning with the right arm) and continue the same exercise 5 times, beginning with the left arm, raising and lowering your body. Concentrate on breathing as frequently as possible during this exercise and vigorously tighten your perineal and abdominal muscles.

➜ You're not done yet! With your knees on the floor, position your pelvis parallel with the floor and keep your body core tight. Stay supported by your arms, with elbows locked and hands positioned beneath your shoulders, your neck stretched out and eyes looking down **(3)**. Lower yourself while breathing in, bringing your chest toward the floor (but not touching it!), elbows bent back and held close to your sides **(4)**. You'll be slightly off-balance, toward the front. Push down firmly on the heels of your hands while breathing hard and contracting the perineum and stomach. Bravo—you now know how to do tricep push-ups!

➜ Start with 3 repetitions of this sequence, and gradually work up to 5.

➜ Relax between the two sequences with your buttocks resting on your heels, your forehead touching the floor, arms stretched out and hands flat in front of you.

Now repeat this exercise every day!

THE + This workout allows you to tone and strengthen the entire body with a minimal investment of time. The stomach, bust, shoulders, and, most importantly, triceps, will all be toned. No more flabby stomach or upper arms. Your figure will be improved and your bust firmer.

MAKEUP TIPS

The right foundation

When we find ourselves looking a bit pale in winter, there's a tendency to use a foundation that's too dark. This is a mistake—it will emphasize wrinkles and add years to your appearance. It's all right to use pressed powder to conceal small imperfections, especially in the T-zone (forehead and nose), and very lightly under the eyes. This is the most delicate part of the face and I recommend a good dark-circle concealer. Thanks to my daughters, I have just discovered Fake-Up Undereye Hydrating Concealer from Benefit, which is excellent.

Don't forget your glasses

Like everyone else, I've started wearing reading glasses in recent years. I'm serenely resigned to this new accessory, but I've had to slightly alter my makeup routine. I suggest that you use a little more makeup on your eyebrows, more mascara to intensify your eyes, and that you emphasize the base of the eyelashes with a black eyeliner pencil to give the illusion of longer, thicker lashes.

My anti-wrinkle egg mask

You don't need a big beauty budget to have lovely skin. Here's a simple, easily prepared recipe to care for your skin and minimize pores. Just combine 1 beaten egg white, the juice of half a lemon, and 1 tablespoon of olive oil. In a few minutes you'll have a rich anti-wrinkle mask. Leave it on your skin for 20 minutes and then rinse with fresh water.

The protein in the egg white is guaranteed to have a lifting effect. Make sure the eggs are organic, of course!

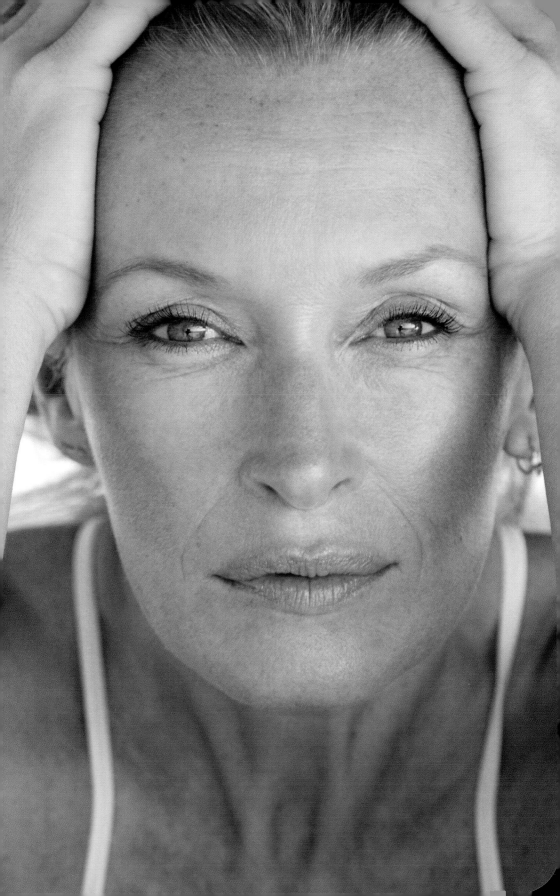

MY FAVORITE THINGS

I am naturally curious and adventurous and I love new experiences and trying out innovative approaches. Here are two of my recent favorite discoveries in the area of health and well-being.

Iyashi Dôme

Have you heard about Japanese infrared saunas?

Like sunlight, long infrared rays are an essential source of energy for the growth of plants and all organic matter. The rays were discovered in the nineteenth century by an English astronomer but it wasn't until the post-war era that the Japanese government began to invest in research to develop a means of regenerating cells. Investigations continue today to explore the action of infrared radiation on heavy metals, weight loss, and overall health.

A half-hour session with the Iyashi Dôme is an excellent way to eliminate toxins from the body. A number of beauty institutes offer this service. It produces the same amount of sweat as a twelve-mile run without harmful effects on the joints.

The Iyashi Dôme appears to be effective, although I'm not convinced of its weight loss advantages. Subjected to heat that is milder than what you'd experience in a sauna, the skin is purified and brightened, and muscle tension and minor pains disappear. It also seems to be a useful treatment for jet lag.

→ Learn more on the website: www.iyashidome.com

Aerial Yoga

Who hasn't dreamed of learning to fly?

The aerial yoga method alternates a variety of movements naturally and gradually, using both ground and air positions.

Practitioners are encouraged to be conscious of their body axis as well as controlling movements and breathing. It's the ideal combination for those seeking both a sense of well-being and the pleasure of physical activity.

A class lasts about 1 hour and each session begins with a period of meditation. The warm-up continues with the initial use of a silk hammock suspended from the ceiling. This is followed by a series of positions based on yoga, particularly the Sun Salutation. The session continues with a muscle-strengthening segment that raises the heart rate before you launch into the air like an acrobat. You'll immediately experience the pleasure of aerial work and feel a sensation of plenitude and fulfillment. The session ends with a period of relaxation.

This method is adapted to all experience levels and is even recommended for people who suffer from back pain and joint problems. I personally love the sensation of being suspended from the ceiling upside down and feeling the blood flowing through my brain.

→ Learn more at www.aerialyoga.com
→ In France, I like the Fly Yoga classes developed by the dynamic Florie Ravinet in collaboration with a team of kinesiotherapists: www.fly-yoga.fr

My seasonal market basket

Fruits
Apples
Chestnuts
Clementines
Kiwi fruit
Lemons
Pears

...

Vegetables
Beets
Brussels sprouts
Cabbages
Celery
Endives
Jerusalem artichokes
Leeks
Mache
Pumpkins
Spinach
Turnips

...

MACHE

Mache (also known as corn salad or lamb's lettuce) thrives in cool weather so you'll find it on festive winter tables, even though these days you can buy it year-round. France is the largest producer of mache, primarily in the Loire-Atlantique region. Originally from southern Europe, it was regarded as peasant food until the eighteenth century.

Rich in beta-carotene and vitamin C—it has three times as much as lettuce—mache is high in fiber and Omega 3 (a rarity in vegetables). Like many salad greens, it has plenty of chlorophyll, which gives the leaves their lovely green color. Often served with beets, mache is delicious in salads. Rinse it first in lots of cold running water but do this carefully as mache is delicate. Season it at the last moment with a mild-flavored oil such as grapeseed or walnut oil.

For a change from salad when the days start to turn chilly, I like to cook mache in a velvety smooth soup.

My Creamy Mache Velouté

5 oz. (150 g) mache, plus extra for garnish
1 potato
1 generous tablespoon of silken tofu
Salt and pepper

Rinse the mache and drain well. Peel the potato and cut into small cubes. Put the potato cubes and the mache in a pot and add 2 large glasses of water. Simmer for about 15 minutes and then blend the vegetables together with the cooking water. Add the silken tofu and season to taste. A few leaves of fresh mache make the perfect garnish.

MY INFUSIONS FOR WINTER

It's simple to prepare infusions. Combine your selected ingredients with fresh water and let the mixture steep in a glass pitcher in the refrigerator.

Apple, Ginger, and Mint Infusion

This cocktail is good for the digestion and works well with both still and sparkling water. Vary the ingredients and proportions according to taste. You can control the spiciness of the drink by adjusting the amount of ginger, which has anti-inflammatory properties.

Blackberry and Sage Infusion

They have a delectable flavor and blackberries also add a bright splash of color to the water. Like all berries, blackberries are rich in antioxidants, fiber, and vitamin C. Sage helps digestion and has a calming effect.

Cranberry and Lime Infusion

The same recipe works equally well with lemons, limes, or oranges. Cut the citrus fruit into slices and combine with cranberries for a cocktail that has a very seductive color.

Cranberries are bursting with vitamins, minerals, and antioxidants.

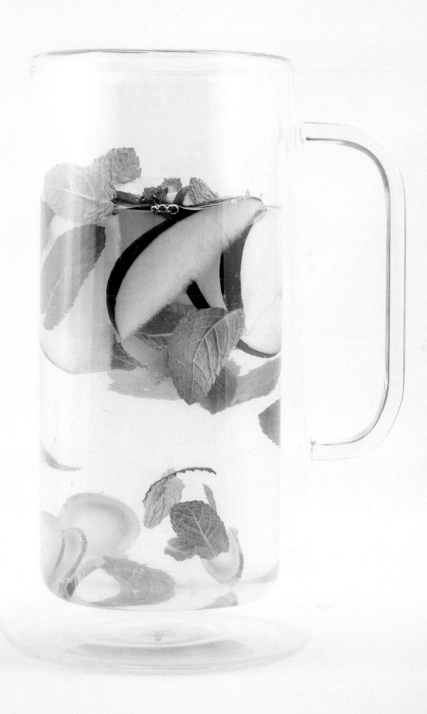

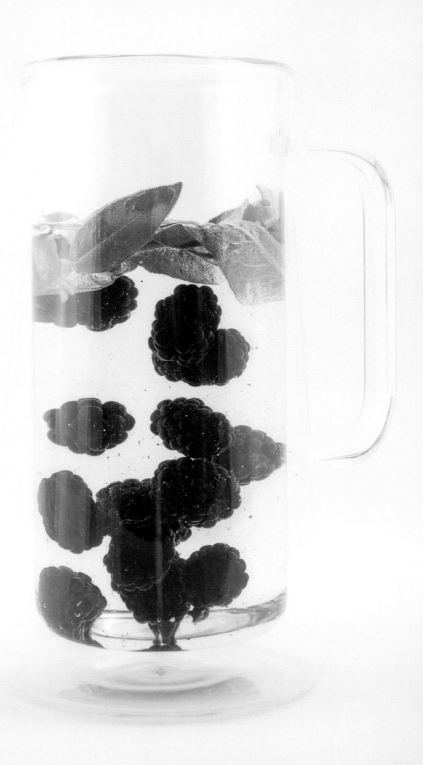

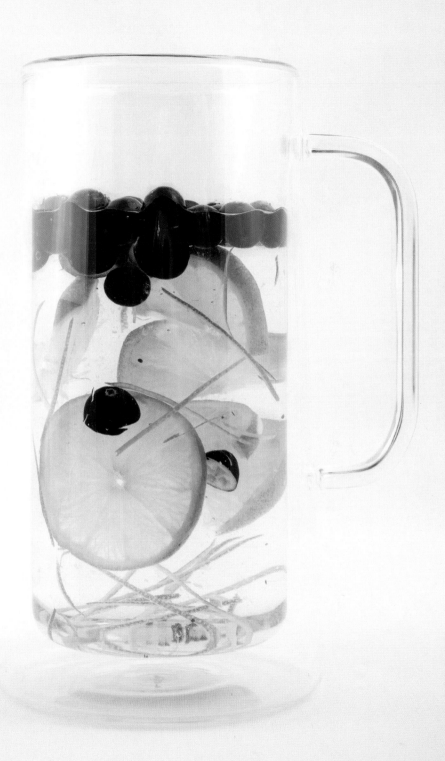

Veggie Curry

Serves 2

Ingredients

2 carrots
1 zucchini
1 red bell pepper
14 oz. (400 g) butternut
squash
1 shallot, peeled and finely
chopped
1 garlic clove, peeled and
finely chopped
7 oz. (200 g) block (firm)
tofu, drained and cut into
small dice
1 cup (250 ml) non-dairy
milk
1 cup (250 ml) non-dairy
cream
3 tablespoons tamari soy
sauce
1 teaspoon curry powder
1 teaspoon ground coriander
Juice of ½ lemon
1 teaspoon finely grated
lemon zest
1 piece of fresh ginger,
peeled and grated
1 piece of fresh turmeric,
peeled and grated
1 tablespoon coconut oil
A few chopped cilantro
leaves
A few coconut flakes

To prepare the curry

Peel the carrots and cut them up.

Wash the zucchini, red bell pepper, and butternut squash and cut into small pieces; discard the seeds from the pepper and squash but there's no need to remove the skins.

Place the vegetables in a pot and add the shallot, garlic, and tofu. Add the non-dairy milk and cream, tamari sauce, curry powder, ground coriander, and then the lemon juice and zest.
Cover and simmer for 30 minutes.

Remove from the heat and add the ginger, turmeric, and coconut oil.
Mix well and serve sprinkled with a few slivered cilantro leaves and coconut flakes.

To boost your intake of vegetable proteins, serve this veggie curry with red lentils.

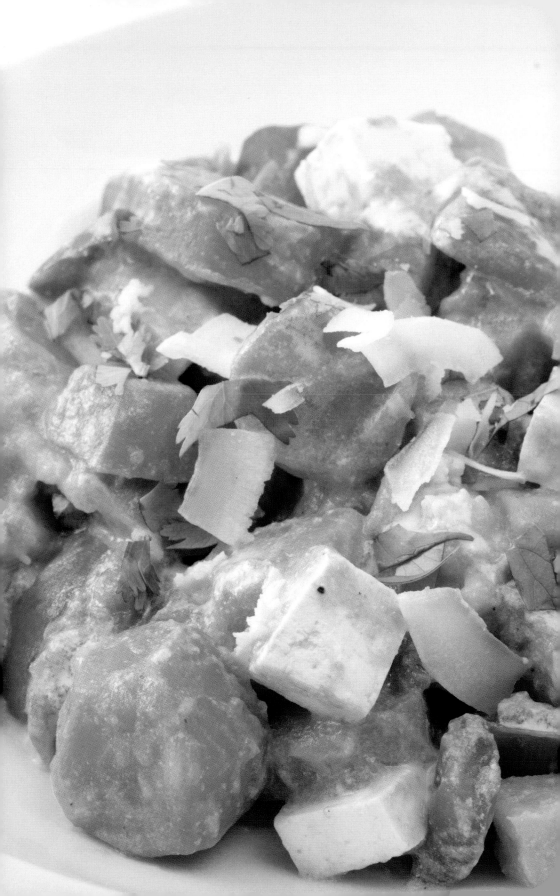

Woodland Risotto

Serves 6

Ingredients

2 medium leeks
2 tablespoons olive oil
1 lb. (500 g) mushrooms, sliced
½ teaspoon fine salt
½ teaspoon thyme leaves
2 garlic cloves, peeled and finely chopped
1 cup (250 ml) dry white wine
Scant 2 cups (350 g) semi-pearled spelt
2 ½ cups (600 ml) vegetable bouillon
1 tablespoon tamari soy sauce
1 large bay leaf
12 chestnuts, cooked and peeled

To prepare the risotto

Cut the white part of the leeks in half lengthwise and then crosswise to create half circles. Place in a sieve and rinse thoroughly.

Warm the olive oil over low heat in a fairly wide, shallow pan. Add the leeks, mushrooms, salt, and thyme. Allow to soften for about 10 minutes. Add the garlic and stir together for 1 minute. Add the wine and simmer for about 2 minutes.

Add the spelt, vegetable bouillon, tamari, and bay leaf. Stir well and re-heat over high heat. Add the chestnuts and mash them in the pan. When the liquid begins to boil, reduce the heat and cover the pan. Allow to simmer for about 30 minutes or until all the liquid is absorbed. Serve hot.

This recipe can be prepared using any type of mushroom. I like to use a combination of wild mushrooms and traditional white button ones.

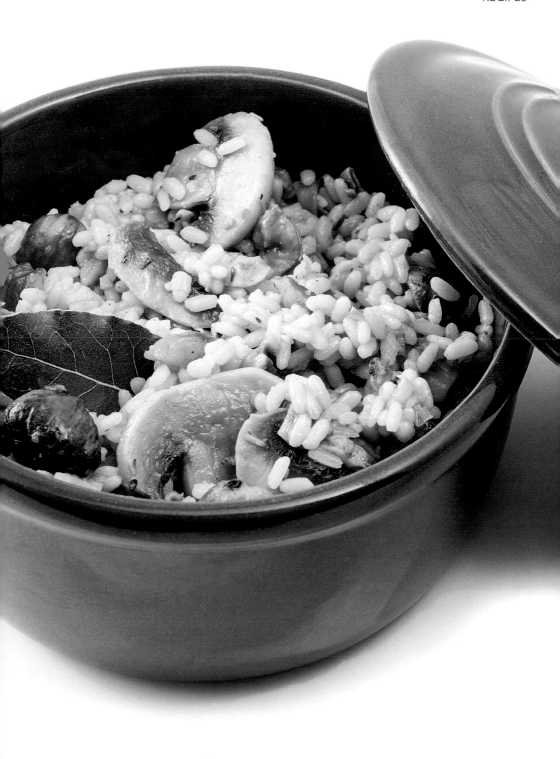

Snowballs

Makes 12 balls

Ingredients
2 cups (160 g) shredded
    unsweetened coconut
2 teaspoons coconut oil
3 tablespoons maple or
    agave syrup
2 tablespoons unsweetened
    coconut milk
½ teaspoon vanilla extract
1 teaspoon ground cinnamon
1 pinch of salt

To prepare the snowballs
Put half of the shredded coconut in
a blender with the coconut oil. Process
at high speed, scraping down the sides
of the blender with a spatula to make
sure the ingredients combine to produce
a paste.

Add the maple or agave syrup, coconut
milk, vanilla, cinnamon, and salt, as well
as a generous ¾ cup (65 g) shredded
coconut. Blend again.

Shape into 12 balls, measuring about 1 in.
(2.5 cm) in diameter, and roll them in the
remaining shredded coconut until
coated.

Chill the balls in the refrigerator for at
least 1 hour. Remove the coconut balls
shortly before serving so they come
to room temperature.

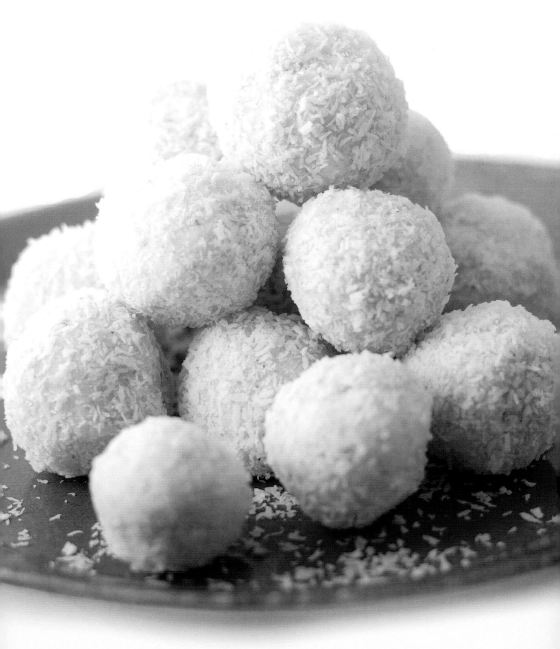

Recipe from Claire Verneil
Pastry chef
Wintertime Sensation

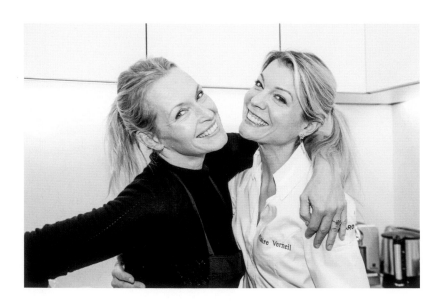

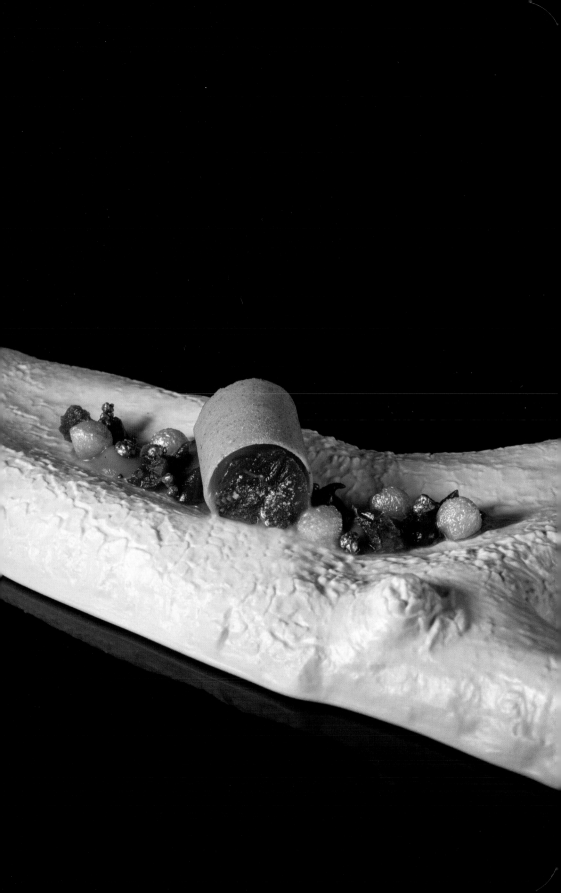

Serves 8

Ingredients
For the gluten-free tuiles
⅜ cup (75 g) cane sugar
1 oz. (30 g) almond butter
1 ½ tablespoons rice oil
3 tablespoons rice flour
2 tablespoons tapioca flour
1 vanilla bean
2 egg whites
Salt

**For the lactose- and gluten-
   free ice cream**
¾ cup (200 ml) rice milk
¾ cup (200 ml) almond milk
2 ¼ cups (400 g) chestnut
   puree
1 vanilla bean
⅝ cup (150 ml) water
5 oz. (150 g) chestnut honey
8 candied chestnuts
   (marrons glacés),
   crumbled

For the pear compote
1 lb. (500 g) Bartlett pears
1 tablespoon lemon juice
1 tablespoon water
4 tablespoons granulated
   sugar
1 large pinch of agar-agar

For serving
2 Bartlett pears
Edible gold powder
Chestnut puree
A few candied chestnuts
   (marrons glacés)
Copper-colored sparkling
   sugar

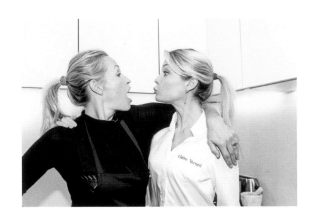

To prepare the tuiles

In a mixing bowl, whisk the cane sugar with the almond butter and rice oil. In a second bowl, combine the rice and tapioca flours and add a pinch of salt. Slit the vanilla bean in half lengthwise, remove the seeds using the point of a knife and add them. Combine the contents of the two bowls. Lightly beat the egg whites with a fork and incorporate them into the mixture with a whisk to make a dough. Leave the dough in a cool place for at least 1 hour.

Preheat the oven to 410°F (210°C/Gas Mark 6–7). Line a cookie sheet with parchment paper or a Silpat sheet. Place a silicone chablon stencil mat, measuring about 4 in. by 2 in. (10 cm by 5 cm) on top and, using an angled spatula, spread the mixture over the mat to make thin rectangular tuiles. Bake the tuiles for about 8–10 minutes until they are golden. As soon as you remove the tuiles from the oven, roll them around a tube mold to shape them into a cylinder. Chill them to firm them up.

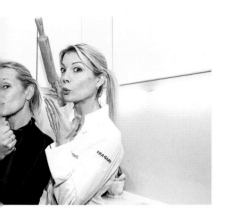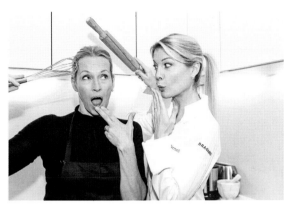

To prepare the ice cream

Heat the rice milk, almond milk, and chestnut puree together over medium heat. Cut the vanilla bean in half lengthwise, remove the seeds with the point of a knife, and add them to the pan. In a second saucepan set over high heat, bring the water and chestnut honey to a boil and continue to boil for 5 minutes until the mixture has a syrupy consistency. Add this to the contents of the first pan and allow to cool. Put the mixture into an ice-cream maker with the crumbled candied chestnuts and churn until thick and creamy. Transfer the mixture to the freezer and freeze until firm before using it to fill the tuiles.

To prepare the compote

Peel and quarter the pears, and remove the cores. Dice the flesh and put them into a saucepan. Add the lemon juice, water, and sugar and cover the pan. Cook over medium heat until the pears are very tender. Remove from the heat and mix together the soft pears with their juice. Put the pan back over low heat, bring to a boil, and whisk in the agar-agar. Remove from the heat, stir, and refrigerate until ready to serve.

To finish and serve

Peel the pears and cut the flesh into small balls using a miniature scoop. Dust them with edible gold powder. Cut 2 candied chestnuts into thin slices and break up the remainder. Spoon the pear compote into four serving plates. Using a small spatula, carefully fill the tuiles with the chestnut ice cream and place a thin slice of candied chestnut at each end. Fill a piping bag with the chestnut cream and decorate with little dots of it piped on top of the compote. Arrange a mini-log of ice cream filled tuile in the center of each and the gilded pear balls and sparkling sugar around the edge. Finish with a few pieces of candied chestnut and serve immediately.

Mindful Beauty

THE BUILDING BLOCKS

Wellness

Health

Fitness

Beauty

Nutrition

Recipes

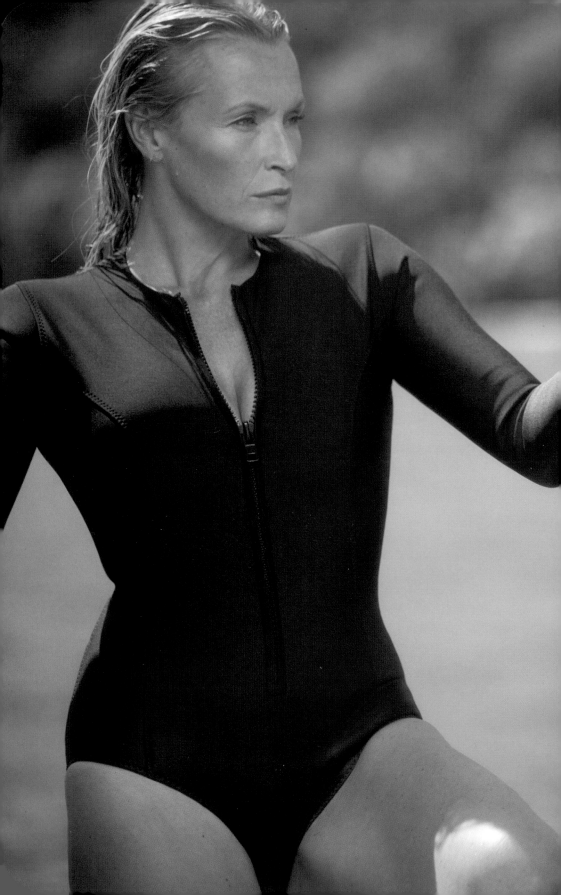

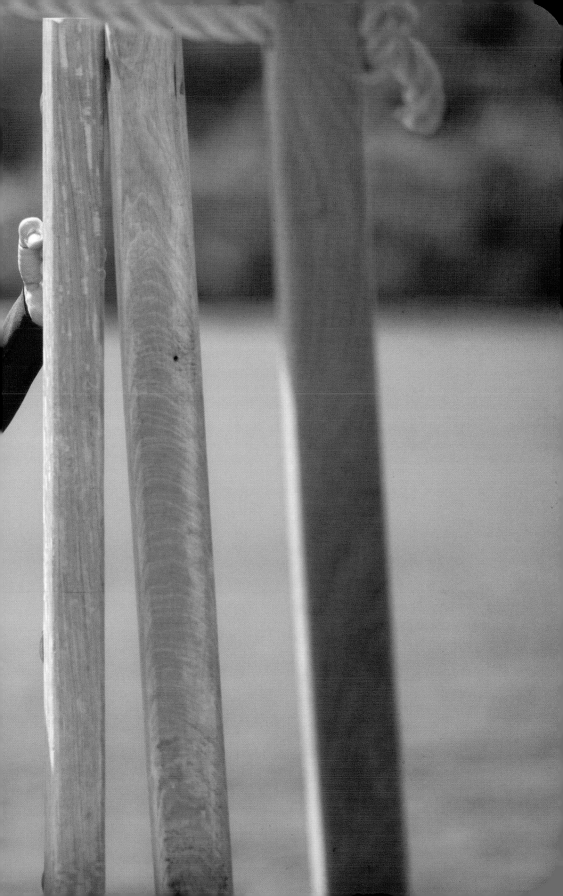

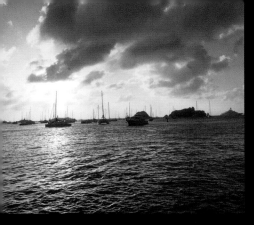
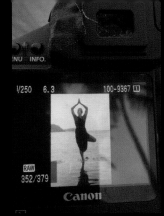
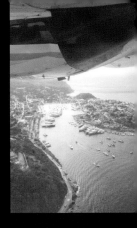
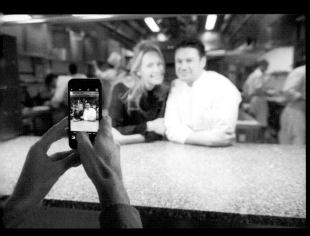
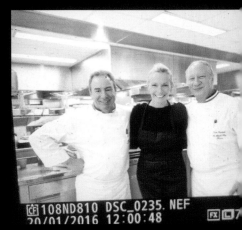
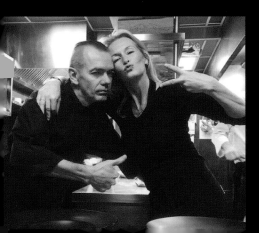
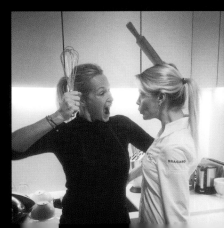
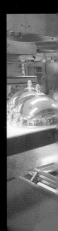

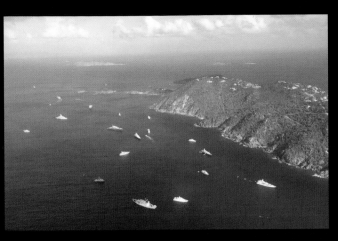
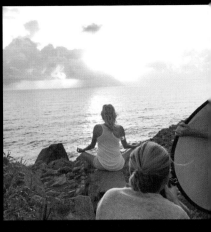
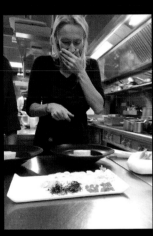
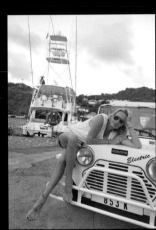
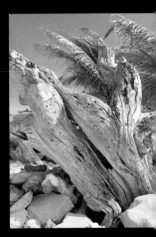
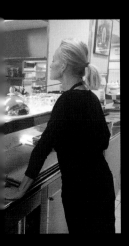
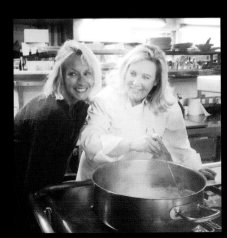
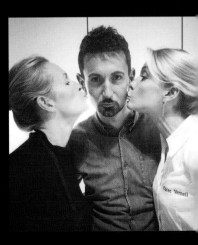

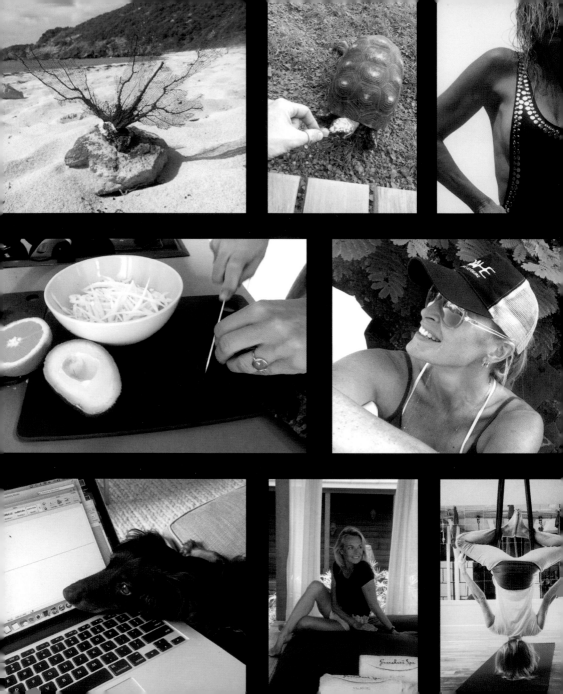

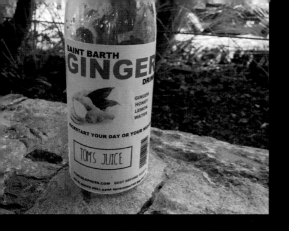
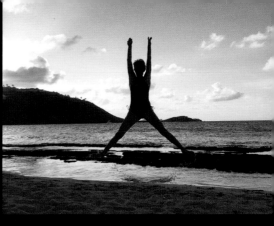

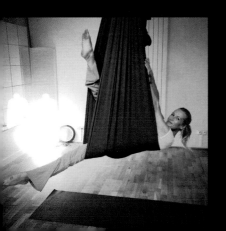
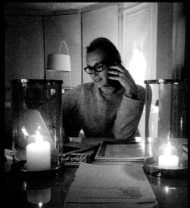
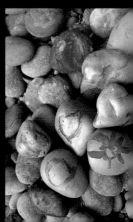

Discover videos, recipes, exercises, and other surprises on **orahe.com**

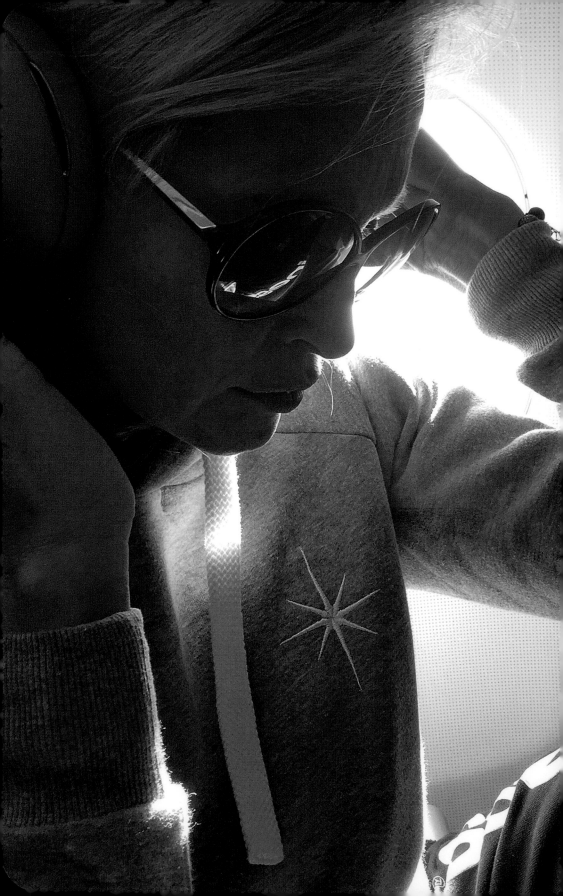

"I don't believe in age—
I believe in energy.
Don't let your age
dictate what you do
or don't do."

TAO PORCHON-LYNCH
YOGA TEACHER, 97

ACKNOWLEDGMENTS

Thanks to my children, family, and friends for their love.
Thanks to Guillaume Robert, my new ally, for his boundless support.
Thanks to Sylvie Lancrenon for knowing just how to make the most of my femininity.
Thanks to Olivier Borde for the superb photos taken in just two days.
Thanks to Aline Gérard for her talent and receptivity.
Thanks to Noémie Levain for her colorful graphic design.
Thanks to Sandrine and Robert Masson for their invaluable advice on health.
Thanks to Julie Laurent-Marotte for her custom-designed exercises.
Thanks to Juliette Poney for her illustrations.
Thanks to Barbara Riera for her time and honesty.
Thanks to Ida at Idalmi St. Barth for providing me with her natural beauty treatments.
Thanks to Claire Verneil for her generous support.
Thanks to Hélène Darroze for her three-star friendship.
Thanks to Éric Fréchon for our Norman collaboration.
Thanks to Alain Pegouret for his generosity.
Thanks to David Faure for his savory extravaganza.
Thanks to Sébastien d'Assigny for his loyalty.
Thanks to Chrystelle Tarreli for her kindness.
Thanks to Ruth Malka for her eagle eye.
Thanks to Olivier Fredenucci for his stylish logo.
Thanks to Christophe Robin for the perfect shade of blonde.
Thanks to Stéphanie Bach and Talos Buccellati.
Thanks to the entire team at the Hôtel Christopher, St. Barts
    www.hotelchristopher.com
Thanks to the entire team at the Hôtel Guanahani & Spa in St. Barts
    www.leguanahani.com
Thanks to Jean-Xavier Favre de Dimco for his lovely table settings.
Thanks to Edmond Lampidecchia of Metro.
Thanks to Virginie Rodriguez of RV Nutrition.
Thanks to Emmanuel Lehrer of Mas de Pierre.
Thanks to Constance de la Fontaine from the Guanahani boutique, to Norma Kamali,
    to Carioca Porto-Vecchio, to Lisa Marie Fernandez, to Wild Side of St. Barth,
    and to Boutique Gisèle for the two-piece Charlie swimsuit.
Thanks to Frédéric Pernelle at Tom's Juice Bar for his vitamin-packed juices.
Thanks to the Ferme de Peyrou for their delicious chestnuts.
Thanks to Gérard Delenne, Les Ruchers du Moulin, for his wonderful natural chestnut
    honey—my favorite.

PHOTOGRAPHIC CREDITS